PRAISE FOR *FIVE TO THRIVE*

"The study of epigenetics is completely changing the way we view disease prevention and treatment. In *Five to Thrive*, information about the epigenetic impacts on cancer prevention is shared with the general public in an easy-to-understand, life-changing way. By describing the epigenetic impacts on five key bodily pathways, the authors are able to effectively teach readers how to use this information to positively transform their health. Tracing the epigenetic impacts of diet, lifestyle, and dietary supplements on cancer prevention is innovative and necessary. This book is likely to help a lot of people."

—*Ajay Goel, PhD, Director of Epigenetics and*
Cancer Prevention at Baylor University

"This stellar book is for all cancer survivors who have asked 'What now? What else can I do?' *Five to Thrive* provides authoritative, natural approaches for thriving after cancer. I strongly recommend this book for all cancer survivors and the people who care for them."

—*Gregory A. Plotnikoff, MD, FACP, Integrative Medicine Physician*
Penny George Institute f⌐ ⁱⁱ   Healing

"This book is not only a passiona'   life to the fullest it is a template for how   venty years, I have witnessed remarkable   ⁱ not teach patients, however, how to trai   .ll of us can benefit from this well researcl   ⌐₁ me influencers of 'vital living.' But for cancer sui   . ..₁yself, this book should be required reading. I have told patients that their diagnosis can offer a blessing of opportunity to enrich every remaining moment of their lives. These authors have blessed us with *Five to Thrive*, a blueprint for building a better life in which we can thrive."

—*Susan W Ryan, DO, Emergency Physician*
Denver, CO, and Melanoma Survivor

"Reading *Five to Thrive* is like having a conversation with a caring and very well informed friend, intent on educating you to make healthy lifestyle changes and motivating you to sustain them. This incredibly valuable resource will serve not only to reduce the risk of cancer and its recurrence, but will also decrease obesity, diabetes, heart disease and many other chronic ailments in those who follow its sound advice. If *Five to Thrive*—with its focus on health and wellness—were mandatory reading, there would be no need for Health Care Reform! I only wish my parents had had access to this information—for their sake and mine."

—*Donald I. Abrams, MD, Chief, Hematology-Oncology, San Francisco General Hospital*
and Integrative Oncologist, with UCSF Osher Center for Integrative Medicine

"Combining scientifically reliable information and compassion, Alschuler and Gazella have created a useful and practical cancer prevention plan. The personal stories from the authors that are peppered throughout the book make it even more interesting and compelling. If you are concerned about preventing cancer, you should read this book."

—*Alan R. Gaby, MD, author of the textbook* Nutritional Medicine

"Destined to become a go-to handbook for anyone interested in improving their health, this book can help diffuse the fears so often associated with the hows and whys of preventing cancer. Amassed with personal insight, experience and dignity, the new work from the desks of Alschuler and Gazella is a must-read for anyone whose life has been affected by the disease."

—*Daniel Rubin, ND, FABNO, Naturopathic Oncologist and Founder/Medical Director of Naturopathic Specialists, LLC, in Scottsdale, AZ*

"Alschuler and Gazella are recognized leaders in the field of natural cancer prevention and treatment. Now, they've distilled all their vital, cutting-edge information about cancer into a simple, easy-to-read book, a must-have resource for cancer patients and their families, as well as those who want to embrace a cancer-preventive lifestyle. Highly recommended!"

—*Ronald Hoffman, MD, Founder and Medical Director of the Hoffman Center in New York City*

"Scientifically sound, and deeply moving, *Five to Thrive* is a rare combination of education and inspiration that motivates and empowers the reader to create the habits necessary to help keep cancer at bay. Nowhere have I read such an in depth explanation of why such things as exercise and laughter affect our risk of cancer so profoundly. The information on how the five pathways affect cancer risk is conveyed in a fun and approachable manner. Congratulations to Alschuler and Gazella for creating a simple, yet comprehensive plan that correctly prioritizes what we all need to do to be healthy."

—*Tina Kaczor, ND, FABNO, Naturopathic Oncologist and Senior Medical Editor* Natural Medicine Journal

"*Five to Thrive* explains vibrant, vital strategies to support cancer prevention. With empowering information and inspiration, Alschuler and Gazella truly guide people to thrive. Follow this path on your journey to greater health."

—*Jeannine Walston, Co-Founder and Executive Director, EmbodiWorks and Brain Tumor Survivor*

"It is so important for people to have trustworthy information about how to lead healthier lives. With a powerful voice of compassion, optimism, and soulfulness, *Five to Thrive* offers just that. Readers will appreciate the wisdom contained in this book."

—*Philippa J. Cheetham, MD, Dept. of Oncology, Columbia University Medical Center, Co-host of Katz' Corner radio show, Medical correspondent for Fox TV*

FIVE TO
THRIVE

YOUR CUTTING-EDGE **CANCER PREVENTION** PLAN

FIVE TO
THRIVE

YOUR CUTTING-EDGE **CANCER PREVENTION** PLAN

Lise N. Alschuler, ND, FABNO,
and Karolyn A. Gazella

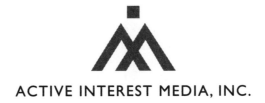

ACTIVE INTEREST MEDIA, INC.

Published by:

Active Interest Media, Inc.

300 N. Continental Blvd., Suite 650

El Segundo, CA 90245

Design by Judi Nesnadny and Karen Sperry

The information in this book is for educational purposes only and is not recommended as a means of diagnosing or treating an illness. All health matters should be supervised by a qualified healthcare professional. The publisher and the author(s) are not responsible for individuals who choose to self-diagnose and/or self-treat.

Library of Congress Cataloging-in-Publication Data

Five to thrive: your cutting-edge cancer prevention plan/Lise N. Alschuler, Karolyn A. Gazella. Includes bibliographical references and index.

Cancer Prevention 2. Health and Wellness 3. Diet and Lifestyle 4. Mind/Body 5. Title

ISSN: 978-1-935297-40-6

Printed in the United States of America

ACKNOWLEDGMENTS

From Dr. Alschuler

I have the unbelievably good fortune to share friendship with some incredibly generous and authentic people. I have also been graced by the presence of bright, compassionate, creative, and smart colleagues. I have the further good fortune of sharing time with people who laugh, play, and revel in life. With a sense of amazed gratitude, I have managed to find a co-author who, in addition to her superb writing, is all of these things as well. I cannot imagine having the fun, insight, revelations, and commitment to the work and spirit of this book with anyone else. Karolyn, I thank you for this most exquisite collaboration.

Fortifying this book with the true grit of vital living are my patients—incredible people who infuse my clinical work and writing with significance and spirit. Your courage, steadfastness, and sense of hope are daily inspiration for me. I thank you for opening up your lives to my scrutiny and for revealing to me your pain, your triumphs, and your aspirations. You are incredible teachers.

In many ways, for me, this book is a tribute to naturopathic medicine. Naturopathic medicine is the well which quenches my thirst for understanding the dynamic forces that shape health and disease. Naturopathic medicine inspires me to remember the beauty and wisdom of the healing power of Nature and the power of the innate healing capacity within every living being. This fundamental perspective has definitively shaped the way in which I understand health and disease.

I would like to offer my gratitude to the scientists and researchers who have dedicated countless hours towards growing our shared understanding of cancer and of health. I rely upon your findings to guide my understanding and, ultimately, to bring wellness into people's lives. Your contribution is tremendous.

I am blessed with a partner who exemplifies incredibly selfless nurturing, unconditional support, and deep rich love. I am profoundly grateful for the gift of experiencing the cozy comfort of daily companionship. Ann, quite simply, the day is complete with you in it. I constantly wonder at how I struck gold with each and every one of my siblings—Britt, Alfie, and Elena. You are all such incredible human beings. This world is a better place because of the service that is your parenting, work, and conscientious living. Mom, you have inspired, loved, and encouraged me always. Your exaltation of the intellect inspires my own curiosity, which I hope to have put to good use in the writing of this book. The pages of this book are once again graced by the spirit of my dad, departed in body, but ever-present in my heart.

Lastly, I thank you, the reader. Where would we be without inquiring minds? It is your quest for learning that fuels our universal understanding of how to lead healthier lives. I honor your dedication to your own well-being.

From Karolyn

Lise you have spoiled me. Writing with someone is not an easy task. But with Lise, it is a true collaboration, a deep partnership, and something I have cherished. It's as if I am writing with a sister who can finish my sentences. To write with Lise is a treat, but to know her as a friend is the real gift. Lise deals with her patients, business associates, and friends all in the same way—with generosity, kindness, compassion, and intelligence. My first thank you is to my co-author, business partner, and good friend Dr. Lise Alschuler, most of all because she makes me laugh.

In the pages of this book (and the last one), there is a name that surfaces frequently, Kathi Magee. She was born Katherine Rose Gazella and our mom named me Karolyn with a K because she wanted some connection with Katherine with a K. While my mom was merely trying to be creative with the names of her only two girls, it's unlikely she realized then that she was creating a connection well beyond the K—and one that would even surpass sisterhood. My sister Kathi is my best friend and she inspires me beyond even a mother's wildest dreams for her daughters. Our relationship transcends blood and is rooted in a deep respect and love for each other that I wish all sisters could experience. I'd also like to thank my sister's main man, Jerry Simonis, who has become a good friend.

I adore my nephews Cody Magee and Travis Magee. You are both amazing, caring young men. I'd like to thank my dad, Don Gazella, and the rest of my family too for their loving support. My life is also blessed by unconditional love from several key four-legged "family members" most notably Beau, Sundance, and Ellie.

Our editor, Deirdre Shevlin Bell, is also a close friend and I appreciate her on so many levels. I continue to be in awe of the kind, nurturing behavior of my friends who are like family to me, especially Maria Dalebroux, Kerrie Moreau, Miriam Weidner, and Susan Ryan. Susan Mesko has also been in my life for a long time and I deeply appreciate her friendship and love. A special thank you to Veronica Smith, who is like a younger sister to me, and her partner Clair Pearson. Also so much gratitude goes to my fun-loving neighbors, not only for their friendship but also for the way they watch out for me: Carrie and Sam Lababidi (and Cody and Jake), Terri and Paul Douglas (and their great kids!), and Cindy and Steve Lowe (and Nana, too). And thanks to my fellow horse loving neighbors Vonda and Alan Kiplinger.

We chose our publisher very carefully and we are thrilled with Active Interest Media (AIM). I have a wonderful working relationship with the folks at AIM, and leading the charge is Pat Fox. Thank you Pat for everything! And a very special thanks to Joanna Shaw who is an awesome co-worker and a good friend. The design of this book was done by Judi Nesnadny assisted by Karen Sperry—what a joy it is to work with you both! Also thanks to Nicole Brechka, Kim Erickson, and our intern Teresa Peterson.

For their talent and incredible commitment to the field of integrative medicine, I would also like to extend special appreciation to my associates at the *Natural Medicine Journal*, Drs. Tina Kaczor and Jacob Schor and the entire Editorial Board. And to my acupuncturist, Jan Vanderlinden, and physical therapist, Sandy Felte—thank you so much for your healing touch. I'd especially like to thank Rachel Naomi Remen, MD, not only for her contribution to this book but more importantly for her contribution to the world.

I end with extreme gratitude for my mom. She is not here and yet she is ever present in my life. She was not perfect, but then again perfect is not always what we need—what we need most often is love. Thanks mom!

PLEASE NOTE

The information in this book reflects the experience of the authors and is not intended to take the place of advice from your own physician. The information is for educational purposes only and is not recommended as a means of diagnosing or treating an illness. All health matters should be supervised by a qualified healthcare professional. You should never attempt to decrease your use of prescription medication without first consulting with your physician. You should also inform your physician of any dietary supplements you are taking. The publisher and the authors are not responsible for individuals who choose to self-diagnose, self-treat or use the information in this book without consulting with their own personal health care practitioner.

CONTENTS

The Five to Thrive™ Plan

At a glance, here are the secrets to successful THRIVING!

DIET
- Engage your senses
- Eat organic
- Whole foods
- More color
- Spice it up

SPIRIT
- Love
- Laughter
- Joy
- Service
- Soul

Transform Your Internal Landscape Through These Five Pathways:

1. Immune
2. Inflammation
3. Hormones
4. Insulin Resistance
5. Digestion & Detoxification

MOVEMENT
- Exercise daily
- Strength
- Stretch
- Cardio
- Nature

DIETARY SUPPLEMENTS
- Omega-3
- Probiotics
- Polyphenols
- Antioxidants
- Vitamin D

REJUVENATION
- Rhythm
- Rest
- Relax
- Replenish
- Rehydrate

INTRODUCTION

THE **PLAN**

"I hate to even think about 'the C word,' but I have to," explained the well-dressed, anxious young woman who approached us after one of our presentations. "My mom had cancer at an early age—actually the same age I am now—and I just started to think about it more."

We hear this sentiment a lot. The topic of cancer is not something we want to think about, but even if we try to shove it back to the dark recesses of our mind it's still there, niggling and periodically poking at us when we hear that someone we know has been diagnosed. At the present rate of diagnosis, one in two men and one in three women will be diagnosed with cancer in our lifetimes. Every 60 seconds someone dies of cancer. It's no wonder it's on our minds.

Rather than let fear rule us, these seemingly daunting odds present an opportunity to take stock of how we are living our lives and determine how we can live better. It is up to each of us to transform that fear and worry into empowerment and zest for life.

"How can I let go of my anxiety when there are such good reasons to be afraid?" a woman inquired after one of our presentations. "Is there really a way to face the threat of cancer and feel good about it?" Her husband put a reassuring arm around her shoulders and hugged her to him. He said, "I certainly hope so, because you and I have a lot of life yet to live together."

For every person confronting cancer, there are several others whose lives are also impacted. We all need to learn how to use this illness, and the fear it evokes, to teach us how to embrace life, meet it head on, and live with vitality.

It is this call for vital living that inspired us to write this book. In the course of our public presentations across the country, we have met thousands of people who share more than the bond of cancer—they share the inspiring drive to triumph over adversity and fight not only for themselves but also for the people they love. We have learned a lot from these courageous people and have also heard their pleas for trustworthy guidance.

This book is a culmination of wisdom gleaned from our own experiences (both personal and clinical), accounts of others who have walked with cancer on some level, and a careful distilling of the research and scientific literature. But most of all, this book is a lesson in *thriving* with a clear picture of what that looks like and how to get there. Thriving is the perfect antidote to fear and the key ingredient to living a vivacious life.

THRIVING VERSUS SURVIVING

Greek philosopher Aristotle once wrote, "The ultimate value of life depends upon awareness and the power of contemplation rather than upon mere survival." The fact that you're reading this book to begin with suggests you just might agree with Aristotle. In fact, few of us are content to just "get by," especially when it comes to our health. And yet when we are in the throes of illness, "mere survival" may be an admirable goal. For some who have battled cancer—or fought alongside a loved one with cancer—simply surviving the fight is success. In fact, we often hear people who have made it through cancer being described as "survivors."

Survivors have emerged on the other side buoyed by love, yet battle fatigued. Facing our cancer fears can create an opportunity to do a deep dive into life to discover its true treasures. Thrivers embrace an intense yearning for vibrant health and vital living.

We know what it's like to move into survival mode. We understand the feeling of taking things one day at a time and, in the heat of battle, appreciating the smallest of victories. We also understand the terror this illness brings. However, it is in those fear-filled moments when we have a great opportunity to achieve a deep awareness of what it takes to effectively transition from *survivor* to *thriver*.

WHY FIVE?

We have a team of people we consult with about our work. We asked our group of loved ones to weigh in about the title of this book and they all loved it. We had already started our Thrivers multimedia initiative (www. Five2Thrive.com), so we knew the "thriving" part was really important to us. But, they asked us, "Why five?" Wow, what a great question! What seemed so obvious to us—the five pathways—was a mystery to others. In the chapters that follow, you will find out exactly how important the number five is to our plan. But here is the short answer.

There are five key pathways that directly influence our health. Dysfunction in these pathways can lead to ill health, whereas optimal function can generate vibrant health—the health of a Thriver! Our Five to Thrive™ plan shows you how to support and enhance the five critical pathways to better health. Our focus is on these five:

1. Immune
2. Inflammation
3. Insulin Resistance
4. Hormones
5. Digestion/Detoxification

While other health plans may focus on one or two of these pathways, our Five to Thrive™ plan is the only program that emphasizes all five. To be healthy—specifically regarding cancer prevention—we must support all five pathways. But how do you do that without being totally overwhelmed? We'll show you.

We applaud your initiative in taking a proactive approach to your health. Our goal for this book is to provide you with a practical, easy-to-use template you can rely upon to help you achieve your highest health goals and to experience life as it is meant to be experienced—with exhilaration and exuberance!

OUR MISSION IS CLEAR

The sidebars on page 11 and 13 explain why we wanted to write our previous book *The Definitive Guide to Cancer*. We have an intensely deep and personal connection to this illness. With *The Definitive Guide*, we chose to focus on integrative treatment because we saw people being forced to choose sides in their treatment—either by conventional physicians warning against natural therapies, or natural practitioners insisting conventional treatment was all wrong. We knew that there was a better way—a way to take the best of both worlds to customize a comprehensive cancer treatment plan. After writing the book, we took our program on the road to various cancer centers, hospitals, and organizations throughout the United States. As we presented our practical integrative plan and heard from attendees, we realized how important it is to apply these concepts and principals not only to treatment, but to prevention as well.

We have written *Five to Thrive*™ specifically for the person who wants to proactively prevent cancer—the person who wants straight answers and clear direction. This book is also for the person who has fought the battle previously and won—and who wants to prevent a recurrence. And this book is also for the person with a family history of cancer, or who has witnessed cancer in a loved one. This book is for anyone who worries about cancer making an appearance in his or her future. This book is for everyone!

During our book tour for *The Definitive Guide to Cancer*, we labeled a book "Thrive" and took that copy to each presentation. Turning the tables a bit, we asked audience participants to sign our book as we signed theirs. Periodically while on the road, we would read what people had written, and it always inspired us. We easily remember the many Thrivers we met along the way. Just being in their presence moved us beyond words. This book and our website are our response to this inspiration. Our goal is audacious, yet simple: we wish to give people the tools they need to take away the fear of a daunting illness and to replace that fear with vital living.

Our book tour schedule was hectic, and at times the flurry of activity would cause us to engage in a frenetic pace that we were not used to. But every now and then, we would be snapped back to the reality of what it means to thrive in the face of illness. Many people stand out, but our experience with one woman was particularly impactful. At our presentation at the University of California San Francisco cancer center, we were signing books and trying to quickly make eye contact with each person as we pushed their book forward in an attempt to move through the long line. As we signed one middle-aged woman's book and looked up to hand it back to her, we both met her emotion-filled eyes. She looked at us and softly said, "Thank you for doing this. I just wish you had gotten here sooner. My husband died three days ago." It took our breath away—quite literally: We both took a deep breath before we gave her our condolences. A moment later, we were once again signing books—but the sharing of her pain had changed us. She is a Thriver in the truest sense. She came to the event—an event she planned to attend with her beloved husband—even though she had lost him just days before. Her courage and steadfast commitment to educate herself and her family continues to motivate us. In her pain, she could have easily given up, but she did not.

Before we ever wrote one word of our previous book, we came together to create a mission and vision. We begin every presentation with this vision and mission and continue to look to these words as our guideposts.

OUR VISION: An integrative approach to cancer prevention and treatment can positively transform cancer care.

OUR MISSION: By educating people with cancer, their loved ones, and their healthcare providers about integrative cancer prevention and treatment, we will reduce the suffering caused by this illness.

Five to Thrive is a natural extension of our life's work toward the fulfillment of our vision and mission. The purpose of this book is to help you prevent cancer and in so doing embrace the potential of your health and your life. We are convinced that the Five to Thrive plan is the most comprehensive, effective way to do that. It begins with a change in perspective and looks at prevention through a different lens.

FIVE TO THRIVE PHILOSOPHY

At the core, cancer prevention is the act of proactively reducing one's risk of developing the illness. But we take our philosophy one step further. To us, prevention means rediscovering vitality no matter what we encounter. The Five to Thrive plan will also make sure you're the healthiest you can be if ever you do develop cancer. It may seem counterintuitive, maybe even radical, to describe a person with cancer as healthy, but the most effective prevention plan needs to also prepare your body for the potential of battle. That prevention plan must provide a foundation for success *against* cancer.

Volumes have been written on how to effectively prevent cancer, and yet we continue to lose the battle and watch people suffer. Why are our efforts failing? According to a survey conducted by the American Association of Cancer Research and the National Cancer Institute:

- Nearly 50 percent of people feel "it seems like almost everything causes cancer."

- Nearly 30 percent feel "there's not much people can do to lower their chances of getting cancer."

- More than 70 percent say "there are so many recommendations for preventing cancer, it's hard to know which ones to follow."

People who are this overwhelmed are often shrouded in a deep fear of getting cancer and end up doing nothing. Here is our response to the survey:

- "It seems like almost everything causes cancer." We will teach you how to enhance your body's ability to detoxify cancer-causing substances and to increase your body's innate defenses against cancer, making you more cancer-resistant.

- "There's not much people can do to lower their chances of getting cancer." We will show you that nothing is further from the truth; the real challenge is selecting the best strategies from among the many available.

- "There are so many recommendations for preventing cancer, it's hard to know which ones to follow." We agree, and that's why we have developed a system that will help you prioritize what you should do from a diet, lifestyle, and dietary supplement perspective. Our system is purposefully simple and straightforward so that you are not burdened with too much complexity in how to live a proactive cancer-prevention lifestyle.

Our plan will help you look at cancer prevention differently. We will show you—based on scientific evidence—that you have the power to change the course of cancer development. At the very core of our plan is the concept of epigenetics, which looks at how we can change the way our genes behave.

We all have cancer cells circulating in our body, yet we don't all develop cancer. Why does one person get cancer while another is spared? This book provides some of the answers to that very complex question with a focus on the exploration and understanding of epigenetics.

Why are most cancer-prevention strategies criticized as being ineffective? Some prevention strategies are not scientifically sound, others are unfocused and do not go deeply enough into how we can physiologically influence our internal landscape, and others are too complex and burdensome to implement. To truly support and transform our bodies on a deep, cellular level, we have found that our focus should be on five key pathways—the very heart of our Five to Thrive program. Scientific understanding shows us that we must address all five pathways if we are to be successful at preventing cancer. These five pathways are:

1. Immune
2. Inflammation
3. Insulin Resistance
4. Hormones
5. Digestion/Detoxification

We are often told that cancer develops as a result of a weakened immune system, yet there are countless people who develop cancer despite having very robust immune systems. We are led to believe that some cancers are caused solely by an excess of estrogen, yet we know this is just one factor. After sifting through the scientific literature, talking to many people with cancer, and evaluating our own personal experiences, we have come to the conclusion that the health and functioning of all five pathways *together* significantly influence the development or prevention of cancer. The key then becomes how we can effectively and easily support **all five**. That's what this book is all about.

Together, we have a combined total of more than 40 years in the natural health industry focused on patient education and patient care, with much of that time devoted to the exploration of the research of integrative cancer care. Based on the scientific literature (and in Dr. Alschuler's case, direct experience with patients), we have been able to narrow down the most effective diet, lifestyle, and dietary supplement strategies that will help you support and internally influence your five key pathways.

But before we dig into the foundational scientific

THE TOP FIVE KEYS TO CHANGING BEHAVIOR

1. Understanding why you need to change
2. Having a plan
3. Not dwelling on setbacks
4. Avoiding all-or-nothing thinking
5. Practicing positive self-talk

---

concept that underlies our strategy—the study of epigenetics—let's discuss the science of something even more foundational: the science of motivation itself. We should recognize what motivates change and how we can ensure those changes become second nature and not a constant struggle.

CHANGE BEHAVIORS PAINLESSLY

The human body adapts to the input it receives. For example, if you normally eat a healthy, organic, unprocessed whole foods diet and then eat several pieces of pizza and a pint of ice cream one night, you will feel the ill effects soon after. However, if you eat pizza and ice cream regularly, your body adapts and will give up sending you signals that those foods are not good for it.

Fortunately, the body adapts just as surely to healthy changes. If you begin walking for 30 minutes four times a week, you will soon notice that you can increase to five times a week and even go a little longer or faster with ease. When walking becomes part of what's normal to your body, it "tells" you when you miss a day. Regular walkers often report feeling tired or lethargic or experiencing headaches, sleeplessness, or anxiety if they miss their daily walks.

Establishing your "normal" occurs in all arenas of self-expression. You can "rewire" your brain to read faster, think more positively, focus more closely, or even become a better listener. You have the capacity to change your behaviors as easily toward the positive as you do toward the negative. With repetition, these new behaviors and thoughts become the new you. The only variable is the amount of time it may take to change that behavior. Some estimates say that in less than a month of doing something fairly consistently, the "rewiring" will be successful and the new behavior becomes a habit. Some research indicates that you don't even have to be 100 percent motivated. Merely wanting to change the behavior about 80 percent of the time will help you successfully transition.

But how do we do this? How do we get to that 80 percent tipping point—and achieve rewiring success? Based on input from a variety of sources, we have developed our Top Five Keys to Changing Behavior. Here they are.

1. **Understand why you want to change.** In the case of cancer prevention, the answer may seem obvious. We want to prevent cancer in order to avoid suffering and untimely death. We understand that cancer prevention may require us to change some behaviors. As you read more, you will be able to identify which behaviors you may need to focus on more than others. Remembering that these changes are the result of our desire to avoid the suffering caused by the illness of cancer is a key motivator to implementing and sustaining the changes.

WHY DO WE FOCUS ON CANCER?
Dr. Alschuler's Personal Connection to Cancer

One of the many gifts I received from my father was the way he approached his life after being diagnosed with pancreatic cancer. Despite receiving the diagnosis along with a three-month prognosis, he stared down the barrel of his remaining life, took aim at the heart of the beast of cancer, and fired. Over the next year and half, he lived his life with exuberance. He learned how to live more healthfully, he repaired relationships, he spent his time with those he loved, and he felt well. One day, as we were enjoying an afternoon on the deck soaking up some delightful springtime sunshine, he turned to me and said, "You know, it has been just over a year since I have been diagnosed. I just want you to know that despite the surgery, the chemotherapy, the radiation, and the clinical trials, I have felt healthier and more well over the past year than I have in the past 10. I don't know if it is all those supplements you have me taking, or my new diet, but I want to thank you."

I was startled to learn about how good he felt. To me he was a constant source of optimism—refusing, for instance, to hear the results of his scans lest his belief in his wellness be contradicted—but I did not realize the depths of his wellness. I reflected on how present he had been over the past year, really living each day as if it could be one of his last. I also thought about the unbounded delight he expressed in seeing others happy, in sharing love with others, in reveling in the very essence of life. I turned back to him and said, "You know Dad, I know the supplements and your diet and exercise are all helping you. But I think they

2. **Have a plan.** Just the desire to change and the understanding about why you want to change is not enough. You must have a practical, easy-to-follow plan that guides your journey. Our Five to Thrive plan will provide you with the structure you need to develop your own health-promotion program. Be sure that goals are realistic. You can always adjust your goals once you are on the path to true change.

3. **Don't dwell on setbacks.** Why is it that we often give more power to the negative rather than the positive? If you eat healthily three days this week, focus on those days rather than dwelling on the four days you did not eat healthy foods.

are helping you so much because of you—you are embracing the very essence of life. You are living fully." "Yes," he replied, "I am dying with my eyes wide open."

Soon after his diagnosis, my father had promised all of his grown children that no matter how long his remaining life was to be, he would live it fully. In doing so, he gave us his last gift—the gift of dying with his eyes wide open. It took a while for me to fully understand what he meant by this, but eventually I understood this to mean using the knowledge of his impending death in order to fully live. He was ultimately successful in giving his children this most wondrous gift, as we were able to witness his courageous, open-hearted, and exuberant living in the face of death. He showed us what it meant to thrive.

It was this inspiration that sustained me through my own diagnosis of breast cancer two years after my father died. Through my own surgeries, chemotherapy treatment, radiation therapy, and hormonal treatments, I also strived to embrace the beauty and wonder of life in and around me. While I certainly experienced the hardships brought on by these treatments, I always felt like a healthy person with cancer, a healthy person receiving chemotherapy, a healthy person receiving radiation therapy. I embraced the integrative approach I recommend to my patients, I welcomed the incredible outpouring of love and support from family and friends, and I let myself dive into each day with my eyes wide open. As a result, I continuously landed in a never-before-experienced place of wellness, vitality, and health. I became a Thriver. This remains my constant mantra: to thrive each day, and to share whatever I can with others so the experience of thriving becomes the new way of living.

Dwelling on the negative simply reinforces those behaviors. Concentrate instead on even the smallest victories. Come up with a mental list of things you did well and think about what allowed you to be successful in those instances. In most cases, lapses are inevitable; however, the frequency and severity of the slip-ups will decrease until finally the desired activity becomes second nature.

4. **Avoid all-or-nothing thinking.** On some level, we have become an "all or nothing" society. Patience is not a modern virtue: We want it all, and we want it now. We also may obsess about doing everything perfectly right now overnight

WHY DO WE FOCUS ON CANCER?

Karolyn's Personal Connection to Cancer

Two days after I turned 33, I was operated on for ovarian cancer. You would think that it would have been the scariest moment of my life, but it wasn't. I was still numb from the events leading up to my cancer. Less than eight months before, my sister was diagnosed with breast cancer. And less than three months before my surgery, we lost our mom to advanced pancreatic cancer. In eight months, cancer hit our family hard. So, while my diagnosis was devastating, I was already severely depressed and honestly didn't really care what happened to me. I had just lost my mom who I adored and a devastating cloud hung over my sister as she recovered. For a time, I wanted to just let cancer take me.

I'm not sure exactly when it happened, but something changed in me. I guess that's no surprise. How can a person go through that experience and not have it change her life forever?

I won't deny that there was a time when I continually looked over my shoulder, just waiting for that nasty cancer to pay another visit. At times I felt helpless, but other times I felt defiant and ready to fight no matter what. Mostly, I fought for my mom's memory and her suffering and for my sister who is a true Thriver. Then, in time, I realized that the fight is much bigger than merely keeping cancer at bay in my body and helping support my sister.

Cancer is a tyrant that has held my extended family hostage for generations. We are one of the largest known families with the BRCA1 as if it's as easy as flipping a switch to instantly change every-thing—our diet, workout routine, relationships, etc. Cancer and cancer prevention are not black-and-white issues and the solutions are certainly not found in an instant. There is a lot of gray, which can drive us crazy, but in this case, the all-or-nothing extremes are not the way to bring clarity. To commit to changing your behavior is to accept the fact that it won't happen overnight. Be gentle with yourself and come to terms with the middle ground.

5. Practice positive self-talk. We could write an entire chapter on the power of positive thinking, but plenty of other resources

gene—the gene that increases risk of breast and ovarian cancer. We have witnessed so much pain and agony associated with this illness that sometimes it's too overwhelming to think about. And yet, my sister and cousins are positive and strong and fight the battle privately with grace and dignity. We have learned valuable lessons from the mothers and sisters who have fought before us. It is because of them that we refuse to roll over and give up.

After our book *The Definitive Guide to Cancer* came out, my sister was diagnosed with cancer again, more than 12 years later. This time the cancer was different and more aggressive. She used an integrative approach—both conventional treatment and natural support—and she remains a Thriver! She continues to inspire me and strengthen others with her positive nature and strong resolve. She is truly an amazing person.

As for me, I have been cancer free for more than 16 years. I still look over my shoulder periodically, but now it is often with a sneer and a flex of a muscle. And yes, there is sometimes a quiet tremble under that muscle. The fear never goes away, but it has moved to the side rather than taking the lead. To live with fear is to be human. One of my inspirations, Rachel Naomi Remen, MD, once told me that fear is not a bad thing; after all, at the heart of fear is the desire to live!

I still remember that feeling of not wanting to live after my mom died when I received my own cancer diagnosis. And it reminds me that my life's goal is not merely to just stay alive, it's to thrive!

already exist on this topic. Our message is to never underestimate the power of positive thinking and to always practice it when it comes to changing your behavior. Visualize yourself being healthy, enjoying healthy food, exercising, and thriving! Surround yourself with positive, optimistic people who will reinforce the healthy activities you are implementing.

Change rarely comes with the flip of a switch. Rather it is gradual, intentional, and sometimes challenging. According to a report in *American Family Physician*, "Behavior change is rarely a discrete, single event; the patient moves gradually from being uninterested (precontemplation stage) to considering a change (contemplation stage) to deciding and preparing to make a change."

Because you are reading this book, it is likely that you are already on this spectrum of change. To ensure that you stay on track, on a separate sheet of paper, think about one area of your life that you are actively trying to change.

Consider the following:

- List some of the things that can get in the way of changing your behavior (e.g., time, money, energy, a certain person).
    - Identify one thing that can help you overcome something on the list you just created and make a commitment to do that by a certain date. For example, if knowledge is getting in the way, one thing you are doing to educate yourself is reading this book.

- If you experienced a setback, identify what that setback was and the circumstances surrounding it. Get it out in the open.
    - What are the situations that may cause a setback?
    - What have you learned from the setback?
    - What can you do to avoid another setback?

- Now focus on the days (or even one day) that you were able to stay the course.
    - Why were you successful?
    - What can you do to duplicate that success?

- Success can sometimes be enhanced by involving others in your plan.

    — Who are positive influencers in your life, and are they aware of your goals?

    — Are there negative influencers who may be getting in the way of your achieving your goals?

    — What can you do to enhance the positive influencers in your life?

    — Can you involve a new positive influencer in your plan (e.g., healthcare practitioner, counselor, family member, friend)?

It's been said the only constant in life is change. That can sometimes be maddening. The key to behavior change is to become attached to the outcome, develop a solid plan, and then be gentle with yourself on days that you fall short. Soon, you will find that the change is complete and you have created an entirely new and healthy way of living. As you embark on changing your life to help prevent cancer and live optimally well, we hope you will find the advice in the coming chapters most helpful.

The next chapter discusses the fascinating, innovative scientific concept of epigenetics. This field of study will completely transform the way you look at health, disease prevention, and even your own body, and will augment your understanding of how it's possible to accomplish the change.

 **HIGH FIVE TIP** *Even if you feel very motivated to become a Thriver, it's best to have a plan that highlights some specific goals. Just as we did before we started writing, why not create a vision and mission statement for your life? Have fun with it! Dream, hope, and articulate what it means to you to thrive. Putting this down on paper makes it more concrete, real, and achievable.*

CHAPTER 1

EPIGENETIC **EXUBERANCE**

T his chapter and the next will take you on a journey into some fascinating and life-changing science. At times it may seem a bit daunting but hang in there! We promise that the understanding and insight you will gain has the power to transform your life into a powerful expression of your greatest potential. Let's begin by explaining epigenetics.

Epi what? What exactly is epigenetics? Simply put, epigenetics examines the idea that environmental factors influence the expression of our genes. Let's think about it this way: Our genes contain the instructions for who and what we are, but they do not function in a static manner. The various traits that characterize each of us as humans, such as having eyes in the front of our head and skin covering our bodies, are the result of instructions derived from genes that we inherited from our birth parents. These instructions are carried by certain genes found within every cell in the body. Yet not every organ in the body has eyes or skin. Why do these genes give instructions to make eyes only in the place where our eyes are located and not, say, on our knees? Because when we were in the womb and developing into a human body, the genes that code for eyes were blocked from being read in every cell except those destined to become our eyes. This example of the selective expression of our genes is perhaps the most elegant and sophisticated display of epigenetics. You—and all other unique beings—are the result of this beautifully orchestrated genetic expression.

Before we delve too much deeper and discover how epigenetics is at the core of cancer prevention, let's review the basics. This may seem a bit technical, but with these basic tools of understanding cancer development, or carcinogenesis, you will have the ability to understand how and why the Five to Thrive cancer prevention program works.

The foundation of epigenetics is the genome. Within each of our cells is a nucleus, which is home to our DNA. DNA is a coiled double helix that contains an individual's genome. The genome is estimated to contain 25,000 to 30,000 genes. Genes are made up of functional sequences of four different nucleotides. The order of the DNA nucleotides determines the message carried by that gene. This message is delivered in a process called transcription.

Transcription, which occurs when the genes are read by an enzyme called RNA polymerase, is the process that cells use to translate the messages contained in DNA into its essential structures and activities. Specific nucleotide sequences tell RNA polymerase where to begin reading and where to end. During genetic transcription, a portion of the DNA helix unwinds, and RNA polymerase sweeps along that strand of DNA reading the nucleotides as it cruises down the strand. As RNA polymerase reads the DNA, it copies what is read and builds its own mirror image of the gene sequence, called messenger RNA (mRNA). mRNA is identical to DNA, with the exception of one type of matched nucleotide. Once the mRNA strand has been completed, it is modified to clip out nonfunctional components of the genetic sequence and is then prepared for the next phase of genetic expression.

That next phase is called translation. The ribbon of nucleotides, mRNA, is fed through another cellular organelle called a ribosome. The ribosome is often referred to as a factory because it decodes the nucleotide message of the mRNA and matches each nucleotide with an amino acid. These amino acids are assembled in the specific order dictated by the mRNA. The formed chain of amino acids folds over itself into unique three-dimensional shapes known as proteins. Cellular proteins form the basis of all of the functioning molecules within cells (e.g., repair enzymes, messenger molecules, growth factors, hormones). Without these proteins, our cells would not function. The types and rate of protein synthesis have a lot to do with the health and function of our body.

Only the parts of the DNA that are unwound and exposed can be read. In fact, most of the DNA in any given cell is not being read at any given moment. The parts of the DNA held in tight coils or with molecules known as methyl groups stuck to their surface cannot be transcribed. Since these genes will not be read, the proteins that are ultimately coded from them will not be made, or expressed. From a functional perspective, this means that only certain portions of our DNA are expressed at any given time in any given cell. And here is where it gets interesting. The environment to which we expose ourselves through nutrition, environmental toxins, molecules of emotion, and other factors can dictate which parts of our DNA will be read. This dynamic silencing and activation of our genes is at the heart of epigenetics.

DNA is a coiled helix wrapped around big proteins called histones. Certain molecules can stimulate an enzyme to cause portions of the DNA to tightly wrap around the histones. As mentioned previously, these regions of tightly bound DNA cannot be transcribed. Other molecules will stimulate a different enzyme that causes the DNA to relax and uncoil itself so it can be transcribed. Like a light switch, gene expression is flipped on when it's relaxed and off when it's tightly coiled. Another way that the DNA can be influenced is when a big bulky methyl group sticks itself to a portion of the DNA.

Just like bubble gum between two pages of a book, this methyl group prevents that portion of the DNA from being read. Another point of influence are microRNAs. These are small molecules that are key regulators of gene expression and primarily prevent genes from being read, often by adding the histones or methyl groups to DNA. Under deleterious influences, key microRNAs are themselves silenced or suppressed, and DNA transcription will be unleashed. This can ultimately lead to uncontrolled growth and cellular proliferation (i.e., cancer). Histone coiling, DNA methylation and microRNA activity are a reversible and dynamic regulatory circuit that controls the expression of our DNA. These processes are under the influence of molecules formed from our diet, environmental exposures, hormonal milieu, and even our psychological state. These external forces have the potential to support or disrupt this regulation. The outcome of these influences on our genetic expression is collectively referred to as our epigenome.

To understand the impact of the epigenome, think about identical twins. Identical twins share the exact same DNA, and when they are born, they are very difficult to tell apart. Even young identical twin children are typically more similar than dissimilar. However, as twins age, differences become apparent. This is most dramatic when one twin develops a disease such as cancer or diabetes, while the other remains healthy. Although the healthy twin may be at increased risk for developing the disease of his twin, it is not guaranteed. That is because the disease is the result of epigenetics.

If, for instance, one twin smoked cigarettes, which contain compounds that switch some genes on and others off, that twin's genome would be epigenetically altered. In fact, cigarette smoke alters the *behavior* of dozens of genes (e.g., it turns off certain repair and suppressor genes). Under the influence of cigarette smoke, cells that are damaged by things such as infection, radiation, or oxidation will not repair their damage, nor will they self-destruct. These damaged cells persist, and yet they don't function properly. Cigarette smoke also switches on some growth promoter genes. When switched on, these genes stimulate many functions of the cell, including cell division. In this scenario, damaged cells, unable to undergo repair, will replicate

(continued on page 22)

EXUBERANCE IN ACTION: ALFRED ALSCHULER *By Dr. Alschuler*

My father, Alfred Alschuler, died of pancreatic cancer at the age of 66. The last year and half of his life was a lesson in exuberance. Not only did he defy his prognosis of three months by living 17 months after his diagnosis, but he lived "out loud" for that period. Although my father would never have been described as meek, shy, or timid at any time in his life, he took his vitality to another level after he was diagnosed with advanced pancreatic cancer. He wrote and spoke about his desire to be "in love with life" and to both feel and express his intense sense of love no matter what physical state he was in.

Throughout the trials and travails of surgery, chemotherapy, radiation therapy, clinical trials, dietary supplements, and ultimately, of decreasing physical capacity, he was ever constant in his exuberant expression of life. This exuberance was manifested in all sorts of ways. Despite having most of his pancreas and part of his intestine and stomach removed in an early, unsuccessful effort to remove the cancer, my father, a great lover of food, continued to happily delight in whatever hearty meal was set before him. He relished in the food because he liked it, but even more so, because he felt that by enjoying the meal, he was partaking in the generosity and love of the person who had prepared it.

My father's exuberance could also be witnessed in his rapturous expression as he listened to one of his favorite classical music CDs— at full volume, no less. The highest points of his day, however, were those spent with members of his family. He had no expectations about what we did together, just that we were together. He spun a cocoon of loving relationships and settled happily and enthusiastically inside.

Although my father was convinced that it was the supplements that kept him alive for so long, I felt it was his exuberance. He breathed life into his genes with the way he loved, and loved to live. He created an internal reservoir of vitality that embraced the life-giving properties of his treatments. I always felt that any recommendation that I offered to him for a therapy had potential, but it was his commitment to being truly alive that gave it traction. My father was amazingly successful in doing this, really to his very last breath. After several days of being unable to speak, and minutes after the last of his children held vigil with him through the night, he took his last breaths. He cried out in a loud and wrenching moan that brought every member of his family running into his room. We all reached out and touched a part of him as he finally took his last breath and, with graceful exuberance, departed this life.

themselves at an increased rate. This, in essence, is cancer formation. The DNA in the twin who smokes is the same as the DNA in the twin who doesn't, but the DNA's behavior is markedly different.

DNA is under heavy epigenetic influence during times of rapid growth, such as fetal development and puberty. Epigenetic mechanisms are necessary for proper growth to occur. These epigenetic influences tend to be quite stable over our lifetime, which is why our eye color, for example, remains the same throughout our lives. While the expression of the genes that code for eye color may not change over time, the expression of other parts of the DNA is altered via epigenetic influences as a result of lifestyle, nutrition, and other factors. Let's look a little closer at how this connects to cancer development and prevention.

EPIGENETICS AND CANCER

In a simplistic sense, cancer is either the result of normal expression of mutated genes or mutated expression of normal genes. In both scenarios, factors external to the DNA change the ultimate expression of the DNA. Let's start with genetic mutations. Some mutations occur spontaneously from exposure to genotoxic agents (things that are toxic or damaging to our DNA). These agents can be environmental pollutants such as cigarette smoke, industrial chemicals, and air pollution. We also sustain genetic damage from our own bodily processes. The normal process of detoxification of chemicals, medications, and hormones generates free radicals, which are highly reactive molecules that will damage DNA unless neutralized by antioxidants.

Even our own hormones, such as estrogen, can damage DNA. Estrogen is metabolized, or broken down, into different substances depending upon which metabolic enzymes are active. Some enzymes, such as cytochrome 1B1, metabolize estrogen into highly active DNA-damaging estrogen breakdown products. Environmental factors like cigarette smoke and certain air pollutants activate cytochrome 1B1. When cytochrome 1B1 is stimulated chronically, estrogen is preferentially broken down into a highly active, genotoxic metabolite. In this situation, our own estrogen is damaging to genes and is generally carcinogenic. Genetic mutations that occur over our lifetime are largely the result of an environmental factor that damages a susceptible area of our DNA. If these mutations are not repaired, and if they occur in a gene that influences cell growth, cancer can develop.

Some mutations are not accumulated, they are inherited. These mutated genes are passed from one generation to the next. Keep in mind that a genetic mutation is different than predisposition. For example, we may be predisposed to a certain illness because of dietary or lifestyle factors that we learned from our parents, but that does not mean that we inherited an actual mutated gene.

Every one of us has some inherited mutations. Fortunately, most of these mutations occur in genes that don't affect our well-

WHY DO HEALTHY PEOPLE GET CANCER?

After most of our presentations, we take questions from the audience. We often receive a version of the same question: Why did I still get cancer even though I had a great diet, I worked out, and I rarely got sick? One audience member in particular was very frustrated as she explained that she was only in her late 30s, had been a runner for years, was a vegetarian, and had no family history of cancer...and yet, she got cancer.

Yes a healthy person can still get cancer. Healthy people cannot exercise or eat away spontaneous DNA mutations from environmental exposures. Healthy people generally have healthy cells with stable DNA, but even then, cells can make simple, yet catastrophic, mistakes in DNA replication, cell repair, or cell division. Healthy people cannot change their inherited genes and, in some cases, cannot effectively compensate for these genetic susceptibilities through epigenetic alterations. While this can be confusing, frustrating, and downright scary, it is important to remember that even though there is no ironclad prevention plan, we can significantly reduce our risk through healthful living. Healthy cells make for hardy DNA, which will provide increased resistance to cancer. Furthermore, healthy people tend to continue to live healthy, vital lives in spite of having cancer. Their prognosis is often better, and they can often manage harsh treatments more effectively.

If you get cancer, it's best to be a *healthy* person with cancer.

being or life expectancy in a significant way. For this reason, we may never become aware of the mutations that we carry and will, in turn, pass along to our offspring. The nature of the mutation varies too. Genes can be composed of thousands of nucleotides. If we inherit a single mutation in a large gene, the change that this mutation creates in the gene may not significantly alter the code for the protein that is ultimately expressed from the gene. These types of mutations, referred to as single-nucleotide polymorphisms (SNPs) are numerous, and we are just beginning to understand their significance. Some SNPs are considered irrelevant to our health and well-being. Other SNPs carry grave significance.

Some of the more well-known SNPs with significant health implications are the inherited genetic mutations to the BRCA1 or BRCA2 genes (see sidebar on page 25). These mutations are examples of SNPs that impair the expression of the BRCA1 or BRCA2 genes. This can have very important health consequences, because BRCA1 and BRCA2 control transcription, regulate cell division, and stimulate cell repair—especially in breast and ovarian cells. Breast and ovarian cells that lack fully functional BRCA1 or BRCA2 are unable to detect DNA damage properly, utilize error-prone repair processes that lead to genomic instability, and divide more frequently. This can result in the development of cancer. While not a guarantee of developing cancer, BRCA1 and BRCA2 mutations can increase the possibility of developing breast cancer to 40 to 85 percent over one's lifetime, depending upon the type and number of SNPs to these genes. Even though these genetic mutations are clear risk factors for cancer, they do not inevitably lead to cancer. Epigenetic factors intervene.

Epigenetic factors can alter the risk of developing cancer, even in the face of genetic mutations. For instance, BRCA1 and BRCA2 mutation carriers who consume the greatest amount and diversity of fruits and vegetables have a lower risk of developing cancer than carriers who consume a narrow selection of fruits and vegetables and consume these foods infrequently. Furthermore, BRCA mutation carriers who prevent significant weight gain during adulthood through overall caloric restriction have lower risk of developing

OUR GENETICS *By Karolyn*

Because both Lise and I have been previously diagnosed with cancer, we are both heavily invested in using diet, lifestyle, and dietary supplements to reduce our own risks of recurrence. This is particularly important given our genetic susceptibilities. Many members of my extended family on my mom's side have inherited mutations of the BRCA1 gene, including my sister. So far I have chosen not to be tested because I live my life as if I do have the gene so not much would change for me.

There have been many breast and ovarian cancers in my family. Given the high incidence of cancer, many of my relatives have elected to have prophylactic (preventive) removal of their breasts and ovaries even though there is no sign of cancer. Due to my genetics, and already having experienced ovarian cancer, I am at extremely high risk of developing breast cancer. However, I have chosen not to have prophylactic bilateral mastectomy. My plan has been to utilize my lifestyle to influence my epigenetics in order to reduce the risk of cancer from BRCA mutation. Many of the preventive strategies that we will be discussing throughout this book are part of my approach. By incorporating these preventive activities into my daily life, I am stabilizing my DNA, reducing genetic mutations, and suppressing tumor-promoter genes. This can go a long way toward compensating for the defective DNA repair BRCA gene.

Although she does not have the BRCA mutation, Lise has some genetic traits that make her susceptible to cancer. Lise has inherited isolated changes in individual nucleotides known as SNPs. Her genetic mutations are located in several genes that make enzymes to detoxify environmental pollutants and breakdown estrogen. As a result, these genes don't work as efficiently as they should, leaving her DNA more exposed to oxidative damage from environmental pollutants. In addition, these SNPs cause her to break down estrogen into DNA damaging metabolites which can be strong drivers of breast cancer tumor growth. While Lise cannot change her genes, she can change her epigenome. She, too, is heavily invested in using the epigenetic strategies discussed in the rest of the book to reduce her exposure to DNA-damaging agents and estrogenic compounds, while switching on her DNA repair genes and switching off her tumor-promoter genes.

To us, epigenetics is not only scientifically fascinating, it's personally imperative.

breast cancer. These findings suggest that epigenetic dietary factors can modify the significance of BRCA genetic mutations.

Another critical link between DNA mutation and cancer development is genomic instability. Genomic instability results from SNPs, from epigenetic silencing of genes that maintain stability, or from significant changes to larger sections of DNA. The resulting instability leaves the DNA prone to mutations. However, epigenetics can influence genetic stability as well. One example of this is a pilot study conducted in 2008 by Dean Ornish, MD, and colleagues, which assessed the impact of lifestyle on telomeres.

Telomeres are protective caps on the ends of chromosomes that lend stability to the chromosome. A chromosome is the linear strand of DNA and the histone and other associated proteins around which the strand is wrapped. Shortened telomeres on the ends of chromosomes cause the DNA to be unstable and are predictive of increased risk of bladder, head and neck, lung, and renal-cell cancers; worse progression and prognosis of patients with breast cancer and colorectal cancer; and increased risk of prostate cancer recurrence. Ornish and colleagues found that after three months of significant dietary changes, meditation, exercise, and supplement use, telomeres lengthened, conferring more stability to the chromosomes. The implication of this is that lifestyle can stabilize DNA, making it less vulnerable to damaging mutations.

The picture that emerges from these understandings is that the interplay between genetic mutations and genetic expression lies at the heart of cancer development. We cannot change inherited genetic mutations. We can, however, utilize our lifestyle to minimize exposure to further mutations and, importantly, to alter how our genes behave. Thus, to understand how to alter our epigenome is to understand how to best prevent cancer.

THE FIVE PATHWAYS OF EPIGENETICS

Epigenetics depends upon the consistency and nature of the epigenetic influences to which our genes are exposed. Let's start with consistency. Epigenetic influences on our genes can be momentary blips—walking through a cloud of car exhaust, for example. The chemicals that you inhale from the exhaust will certainly influence the behavior of your genes, but the influence will be short-lived and ultimately not likely to be impactful in a long-term way. What happens though if you live near a busy intersection, walk to work along major roads every day, and work in a busy city? Now your exposure to the chemicals in car exhaust is daily and long-term. This is when the epigenetic influences exerted by these chemicals begin to make an impactful difference in how your genes behave.

Aside from the time we spent in the womb, epigenetic changes tend to accumulate over our lifetime. This means that epigenetics is the result of daily habits and exposures over months and years that create sustained changes in how our genes behave.

Our genes' behavior will only change if external influences are translated into molecular events around our DNA. This translation occurs via key bodily pathways. In fact, there are five key bodily pathways that are responsible for the vast majority of this translation. Understanding the link between the health of these pathways and our epigenome is at the heart of understanding our effective cancer prevention program.

Our genes exist within a dynamic molecular soup. The molecules floating in and around the DNA can influence the DNA "switches" and turn on or off certain genes. Thus, epigenetics is the result of the molecules to which the DNA is exposed. Just as the flavor of soup changes depending on which ingredients are added to the broth, the nature of epigenetic changes is dependent upon the molecules that consistently interact with our DNA.

The most powerful determinants of these molecules are the five key pathways of immunity, inflammation, insulin resistance, hormonal balance, and digestion/detoxification. The health and functioning of these pathways yield molecular changes that can dramatically affect the expression of our genes. It is for this reason that improving the health of these five pathways is so critical to cancer prevention. Chapter 2 describes each of these pathways and their key epigenetic influence points. Every cancer prevention strategy that we outline in this book ties back to improving health through one or more of these key pathways. This is significant because it is how we influence our genes.

Preventive strategies work because they are translated through our key pathways to cause predictable changes in our cellular environment. These internal environmental changes, in turn, turn off cancer-promoter and cell-proliferation genes and turn on cell-repair genes. Using our lifestyle to influence the health of our key pathways in order to change our internal molecular environment can switch on protective genes and switch off tumor-promoter genes. Over time, this will lower our risk for cancer, along with other major illnesses like heart disease and diabetes.

EPIGENETIC EXALTATION

All of this is really cause for celebration. Our genes are not our destiny. We have the opportunity, through the choices we make, to change our genetic expression. Much like the musical notes on a page, the music that is us depends entirely upon how the notes are played. While we cannot change our internal notes, we can play some loudly and others softly, and we can repeat some and skip others, changing the song completely. This gives us tremendous opportunity to alter our genetic destiny, but it's also a huge responsibility because it means our choices have repercussions that affect us down to our genetic core. It is our hope that when reading the coming chapters, you will gain motivation and direction to influence your genes toward the healthiest you possible—toward your own epigenetic exuberance!

 **HIGH FIVE TIP** *Lifestyle is an epigenetically powerful tool that can put the brakes on cancer. While cancer may be the result of injured genes, we have the ability to alter the expression of genes over our lifetime and, in so doing, to minimize the risk of cancer. The key to success lies in practicing healthy habits over your lifetime. It is the repetition of good health that resists cancer.*

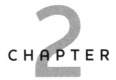

CHAPTER 2

MEET THE **PATHWAYS**

ancer is very cunning. We need a prevention plan just as crafty and even more powerful than cancer itself. The key to cancer prevention involves training our cells to retain their optimal resistance and effectiveness over cancer while also creating an environment that is inhospitable to cancer growth. And, that is where the five pathways play a pivotal role.

While cancer can be daunting, the good news is that the human body is actually well equipped to fight cancer. We have biological pathways designed to keep us healthy and cancer-free. In fact, our bodies are designed with many cancer prevention tools already in place; we just need to learn how to use them and use as many as possible. We may have strong immunity, for example, but what about our detoxification system? Cancer uses a multifaceted approach to survive, and we need to do the same to prevent it. Focusing on one aspect of prevention is shortsighted and ineffective. It's not just one *thing* that causes cancer, and it's not just one *thing* that prevents it.

For those people diagnosed with cancer even though they were fairly healthy, we ask them to look at all of the five key pathways just as we have in our own individual circumstances—immunity, inflammation, insulin resistance, hormonal balance, and diges-tion/detoxification. Using the pathways to help us prioritize also helps us determine the most critical components of an individual-ized prevention plan. This means thinking about how to use diet, lifestyle, and dietary supplements to properly support each path-way. There are practical, simple ways to do this. Before we show you how to support the pathways, let's first take a look at the form and function of each of the five.

BACTERIAL FRIENDS AND FOES

We are made up of about 100 trillion bacteria. Bacteria actually out-number our cells by 10 to 1, so we are more bacteria than we are cells! Fortunately, most of those bacteria are friendly and work hard on our behalf. The majority of friendly bacteria we carry around live in our intestines. They coat the intestinal lining to help prevent toxins and large food particles from entering the bloodstream. Friendly bacteria also aid in digestion, produce vitamins and energy for the body to use, and support a virulent immune system.

There are several factors that can destroy friendly bacteria and cause harmful bacteria to grow out of control. Some of these include:

- Antibiotic use
- Poor diet
- Lack of exercise
- Increased stress

An imbalance of bad to good bacteria can cause a number of problems, including a weakened immune system. Friendly bacteria must be continually replaced and supported. You can do this with a healthy diet and increased activity levels, but we also recommend taking a probiotic dietary supplement on a daily basis. We'll discuss the value of probiotics more in chapter seven.

1. IMMUNE

You may think our knowledge of the human immune system would date back centuries, but that's not the case. Most of what we know about how the immune system works and how to enhance and protect it is only decades old. A great deal remains to be discovered. But what we do know so far gives us ample opportunity for making improvements.

When the immune system is functioning properly, it is the most complex and intricately choreographed dance of life that you can imagine. The first step of our immune dance is to identify antigens. Antigens are tags on mutated cells (cancerous cells) and invading microorganisms that immune cells, namely macrophages and dendritic cells, recognize and process into signals for other immune cells. This is known as antigen sampling. Upon sampling these tags, the macrophage or dendritic cell is able to determine whether the cell or organism is normal and can stay or is abnormal and requires removal. Macrophages and dendritic cells can be thought of as the roving eyes of our immune system because they are constantly on the lookout for foreign antigens as they circulate throughout our bodies.

Once a macrophage or dendritic cell samples and processes an antigen and determines it to be dangerous, it presents this information to another immune cell, the helper T cell, which releases molecular messages known as cytokines. These cytokines direct the aptly named killer T cells and natural killer (NK) cells to destroy any cell expressing this antigen. Killer T cells and cytotoxic NK cells inject the mutated cells with toxic compounds and cause the cells to die. The dead cells are completely digested by the cytotoxic T cells and thereby eliminated from the body. The most fascinating aspect of that entire process is that it happens in an instant and it happens constantly!

Here are some interesting questions to ponder about immunity:

- **Why does the antigen processing even involve the helper T cell?** Why doesn't it just go directly to the killer T cell? There are helper T cells in the body that actually store information about these antigens just in case they encounter them again. This cellular memory is brilliant because it helps the immune system respond even faster the next time it encounters that type of antigen. Plus, the helper T cells play a critical role in directing the cytotoxic T cells to the antigen-bearing cancer cells.

- **How do all these immune cells do this so quickly?** Immune cells circulate within the extensive channels that make up our lymphatic system, and some reside in the extracellular fluid that bathes our cells. This means our specialized immune cells can be rapidly mobilized to wherever they are needed.

- **What happens if the immune cells make a mistake and label a good cell as an antigenic cell?** This actually does happen and is known as an "autoimmune" response—the immune system tags healthy cells for destruction. Examples of autoimmune conditions in which this self-directed immune response is ongoing are rheumatoid arthritis, Crohn's disease, type 1 diabetes, and lupus.

- **How does the immune system prevent an autoimmune response from occurring?** The immune system has suppressor cells called regulatory T cells. These immune cells inhibit the activity of T cells, effectively shutting down an immune reaction. This is a critical check in our immunity's check-and-balance system. Unfortunately, in the case of cancer, tumors hijack this process by secreting large amounts of chemicals that recruit regulatory T cells to the area of the tumor. Tumors shield themselves with regulatory T cells, which essentially shuts down the cytotoxic immune response to those cancerous cells.

As you can see, the immune system is like a group of finely choreographed dancers, responding to threats in a precisely coordinated manner. The strength of our immune system comes from the actions of each of its members as much as the coordinated efforts of them all. The most important thing to remember is that both of these aspects can be influenced epigenetically. For instance, mushrooms and yeast extracts contain compounds called beta-glucan polysaccharides that increase NK cell activity by activating certain genes in those cells. Mushroom-derived polysaccharides also decrease genetic expression of Transforming Growth Factor-beta (TGF-beta), an immunosuppressive cytokine secreted by T regulatory cells.

Another example of how we can influence the behavior of the genes in our immune cells comes from research on mindfulness-based stress reduction. Mindfulness-based stress reduction originates from Eastern meditation practices and cultivates conscious awareness in a non-judgmental manner. Several small trials have shown that mindfulness-based stress reduction, and meditation in general, improves immunity, especially increasing NK cell activity via genetic activation of certain cellular pathways. Increased NK cell activity is associated with increased disease-free survival in many human cancers.

The immune system is a complex, sophisticated example of the power of the human body. Supporting this amazing internal defense system is incredibly important when it comes to preventing cancer. Interconnected with the immune system is the process of inflammation. The inflammatory pathway is often misunderstood—and certainly underestimated—when it comes to its role in cancer.

2. INFLAMMATION

A bump on the head will result in swelling and bruising. This is our inflammatory response in action. When we think of inflammation, we think of that bump on the head, a swollen joint, or an irritated infection. We rarely think of cancer. However, research shows that an overactive, continual internal inflammatory response can directly cause cancer. Before we explain that link, let's take a closer look at what's going on when something is inflamed.

The same warriors of the immune system that kill antigenic cells also initiate inflammation. When you bump your head, white blood cells and antibodies are sent to the spot to help filter out bacteria and debris. A type of white blood cell known as a neutrophil will remove these foreign particles by eating them. This can take some time, so reinforcements known as macrophages (literally meaning "big eaters") often are sent to help in the clean-up process. Lymphocytes will also join the effort. The lymphocytes send messages to the immune system with updates. Depending on the progress, the immune system will either continue the effort or stop the process.

When you see the redness and swelling of a bump or injury, think of all those hard-working inflammatory cells in action. The increased blood flow to the area can cause tissues to puff up, which can then compress nerve endings. That's why sometimes we have pain associated with an inflammatory situation. The immune cells responding to the injured tissue secrete molecular messages throughout the process. These messages stimulate cells such as fibroblasts, the construction workers of our body, to lay down the scaffolding for new tissue. The immune messages call out for blood vessels, bringing needed nutrients into the area. These messages also increase the rate of cell division so the tissue can knit itself together more quickly.

In the case of a bump or cut, this is exactly the type of response we want. It's a surge of controlled activity allowing our body to wall off the injured area and rapidly repair the tissue. But what happens when, instead of a bump or bruise, the inflammatory process is initiated by an injury that is perpetual such as exposure to environmental pollutants or even nutrient deficiencies? This can create an inflammatory cycle that continues well past the time of the acute exposure. This chronic internal inflammation can increase our risk of developing cancer.

Most of us, as we age, become chronically inflamed, at least to some degree. The ravages of daily living take their toll on us over the years, leaving us in a perpetual state of inflammation. In many ways, chronic inflammation is the manifestation of a multitude of factors that can eventually overwhelm the set points of our cells and tip them toward overproduction of inflammatory molecules.

The main trigger of inflammation is oxidative damage to our cells. Oxidative damage is the result of a chemical reaction to various cell-damaging agents. For example, ultraviolet radiation from the sun, industrial pollutants, and cigarette smoke cause oxidative damage to our cells. Interestingly, some activities essential to life also produce oxidative damage, such as breathing, exercise, and eating. All of these oxidative triggers require an antioxidant response in order to prevent tissue damage and inflammation. This antioxidative response, in turn, requires that we keep our cells well supplied with antioxidant nutrients from the diet, and that the antioxidant stores in our bodies are well supported with sleep and relaxation. As mentioned in the sidebar on page 35, if our antioxidant "bank" becomes depleted, cellular oxidative damage will get the upper hand. If left unchecked, oxidative damage results in inflammation that over time will cause tissue damage and contribute to diseases such as cancer.

OXIDATION AND ANTI-OXIDATION

What happens when you cut an apple in half and let it sit out for a few minutes before you eat it? It turns brown. This is oxidation. It's the same process that causes an avocado to turn black, a car to rust, and copper to develop a pretty patina. The simple process of oxygen interacting with other molecules in fruits, vegetables, metal, and even the cells in your body, causes a reaction. In some cases, like that rusty car or the copper roof, this process can take a long time. In other cases, like with the apple, the process can occur pretty quickly.

Oxidation technically means the loss of at least one electron from a molecule's orbiting cloud of electrons. This missing electron is very destabilizing to the molecule and leaves it hungry for another electron to replace what it lost. This unstable, highly reactive molecule is called a free radical. Picture a plane with only one wing or a boat that's lost its rudder. Those are great visuals of a free radical—out of control. In the body, free radicals spin out of control looking for that missing electron. In the process, they can do a lot of damage. What's worse is that free radicals are formed constantly. After we exercise, if we are fighting an infection, and even after we eat a meal, free radicals are created. We can visually see free radical damage as we age in the form of wrinkles on our skin. How do we overcome this harmful process that results from everyday oxidation? Antioxidants!

The human body is designed to keep free radicals in check. We have an internal antioxidant "bank" and we make "deposits" with the foods we eat. These antioxidants help us quench free radicals. The problem occurs when the diet is low in antioxidant-rich foods such as fruits and vegetables, or if we are exposed to an increased amount of free radicals through pollution, stress, or excess chemicals in our foods. When our antioxidants can't keep pace with our oxidants, free radicals are formed and tissue oxidation occurs. This is a highly inflammatory process. This means you need to make constant deposits to your internal antioxidant bank. You can do this by eating a diet of fruits and vegetables, reducing processed foods, and taking antioxidant dietary supplements. (You will find more information about dietary and supplemental antioxidants in Chapters 5 and 7.)

The molecules of inflammation are designed to stimulate tissue repair by increasing cell growth and the flow of nutrients into the area. This works well for acute healing, but can wreak havoc long term. Nowhere is this more problematic than in the presence of a damaged cell. Inflammation drives cell growth and if the cell that is dividing is a damaged one, this can lead to the development of a tumor. Chronic inflammation creates the perfect road for damaged cells to travel, and the eventual destination can be cancer.

While cancer growth can result from chronic inflammation, cancer can also initiate and perpetuate inflammation. When a mutated cell divides, it passes its mutations to the next generation of cells. With each round of cell division, the population of mutated cells grows, and soon a little colony of mutated cells exists. The body responds to these cells as it would any other invading or foreign compound—with an inflammatory response. The problem is that by the time cancer cells are collected into a colony, they are pretty good at evading immune detection and destruction. Thus, the growing tumor acts like an unhealed wound that continually triggers an inflammatory response.

The main inflammatory responder is a protein known as nuclear factor kappa B (NF-kB). NF-kB is the king of our inflammatory response. Once it is activated, it directs a series of events that culminate in inflammation. Under "the king's" direction, cell division is stimulated, ostensibly to help injured tissue repair itself. NF-kB also stops cells from killing themselves—a process known as apoptosis—so that the cells persist longer in order to support the tissue's response to the injury. Under NF-kB's command, many genes that code for various other inflammatory molecules are activated.

These other inflammatory molecules include COX-2 enzymes and powerful cytokines such as interleukin-1 (IL-1), interleukin-6 (IL-6), and interleukin-8 (IL-8). The result is an elite messenger corps that diffuses into injured tissue and activates numerous other events, thus helping to perpetuate the inflammatory response. Blood vessels are called in, cell division is up-regulated, and the activity of certain genes is increased. When NF-kB is activated, so is the entire inflammatory "kingdom". This amplified inflammatory response is perfectly suited to a localized injury or infection. However, if the inflammatory trigger is a colony of cancer cells, this inflammatory reaction can be very problematic.

The cancer cells respond to these inflammatory molecules similarly to how healthy cells react. Thus, in the presence of NF-kB and its downstream inflammatory cytokines, cell death (including cancer cell death) is *decreased*, and cell division is increased. Increased cell division of cancer cells is not a good thing. Unfortunately, cancer cells, unlike an injury or infection, do not heal in an inflamed environment. Instead, because it is acting like an unhealed wound, cancer continues to trigger this inflammatory cascade. This prolonged response ends up doing exactly the opposite of what we want when we are trying to prevent cancer, as NF-kB and its collaborators, COX-2, IL-1, IL-6, and IL-8 disrupt the checks and balances that control cell growth and activity. High blood levels of IL-6 is a prime example of an inflammatory molecule that perpetuates cancer growth and that is:

- correlated with shorter survival among women with advanced breast and ovarian cancers;

- associated with shorter survival in patients with leukemia, as well as kidney and prostate cancers; and

- linked to growth and invasion of breast cancer cells.

In addition, elevated IL-6 corresponds with the release of another harmful molecule known as vascular endothelial growth factor (VEGF). VEGF increases blood supply to tumors—which is harmful because cancer needs a reliable blood supply in order to survive.

Whether chronic inflammation is due to cancer or to other oxidative damage, we know that it can sustain cancer's growth. Thus, a significant factor in impeding cancer's growth lies in our ability to quench the inflammatory embers before they become forest fires. Inflammation is our body's call to action. But if left unchecked, it can contribute to a number of illnesses, including cancer, arthritis, dementia, diabetes, and heart disease. And the longer the inflammation persists, the higher the risk of developing these illnesses. Cancer cells are opportunistic and ready to take advantage of an environment that allows them to multiply and invade easily. Fortunately, through harnessing the power of epigenetics, we can change the course of chronic inflammation.

Diet has a huge influence on the expression of inflammatory genes. For instance, consumption of saturated fat (found in red meat, dairy products, and fried foods) results in increased expression of genes involved in inflammation, whereas monounsaturated fat (olive oil) consumption leads to a more anti-inflammatory gene expression profile. Another powerful way to reduce inflammation is to consume flavonoids. Flavonoids are the pigmented compounds that give hue to the beautiful array of colored fruits, vegetables, and spices we eat. These flavonoids are also potent anti-inflammatory molecules. The naturally occurring flavonoids found in turmeric (curcumin), resveratrol from red grape skins, and epigallocatechin gallate (EGCG) from green tea, among others, directly scavenge free radicals, down-regulate NF-kB and other signaling pathways, and up-regulate anti-inflammatory pathways, such as glutathione synthesis. The net antioxidant and anti-inflammatory effect of these foods can epigenetically alter the course of chronic diseases. We discuss this concept in much more detail in Chapters 5 and 7.

So far we have discussed the importance of a strong immune system and a controlled inflammatory response; both pathways need the proper balance to function effectively. But the pathway with the most fragile balance is our endocrine system, where hormonal harmony is paramount for optimal cancer prevention.

3. HORMONAL BALANCE

The endocrine system may not get a lot of your attention when compared to your heart, brain, or immune system, but the organs and glands of the endocrine system significantly contribute to growth and development. These glands are major influencers of all other systems and are strategically placed throughout the body. They include:

- Pituitary and pineal (in the brain)
- Thyroid and parathyroid (in the front of the upper part of the throat)
- Thymus (in the front of the chest, above the heart)
- Pancreas (behind the stomach; connected to the beginning of the intestine)
- Adrenals (one on top of each kidney)
- Ovaries and testes

These glands secrete hormones, which are powerful messenger molecules that help regulate body systems and functions, including:

- Calcium uptake by cells for strong bones
- Heart rate and blood pressure
- Immune response
- Breathing
- Secretion of digestive enzymes
- Blood sugar regulation
- Brain function
- Development and function of reproductive organs
- Metabolism and energy levels

As you can see, hormones are very diverse and powerful. We need hormones to do even basic things that we take for granted, like breathing. Hormonal activity has far-reaching effects throughout the entire body. Think of the endocrine system as a beautiful garment. What happens if you pull on a loose thread of that garment and keep pulling? The garment will unravel, right? The interconnectedness of our entire endocrine "garment" requires constant resetting and rebalancing. This interconnectedness also means that chronic internal stress on a portion of the endocrine system will have a profound unraveling effect on other body systems, such as immunity and digestion. The keys to the endocrine system are balance, rhythm, and a scientific term known as homeostasis (maintaining that dynamic internal equilibrium). But how does hormonal balance relate to cancer prevention?

The link between hormones and cancer goes beyond the obvious hormone-dependent cancers such as breast, ovarian, and prostate. Given the powerful, extensive effects of hormones as described previously, it makes sense that hormonal balance can influence the growth of cancer cells as well as other cells. All cells, including cancer cells, have hormone receptors. No matter where the cell is located, it receives a message when the matching hormone attaches to the cell's receptor—and most often, that message is to grow and divide.

It may sound like an alien movie, but hormone receptors are sophisticated, complicated structures that create very specific pockets. Only certain messengers can fit into these pockets, making the receptors extremely picky about what molecules will trigger a specific action. Once a molecule fits into this pocket, the entire receptor changes shape, which initiates other events inside the cell membrane, ultimately sending a succession of signals all the way to the DNA.

To better understand how these receptors work, think of the receptor as a lock in a door, and think of the circulating hormone as the key. As the hormone (the key) circulates, it's looking for the right lock (receptor). If the hormone fits into the receptor, it "unlocks" the lock and "enters" the cell. More precisely, this unlocking process initiates a cascade of activity that ultimately alters the behavior of the cell. Receptor-stimulated activity controls an enormous number of critical cellular functions. This is a good thing, for example, if it is a bone cell and the unlocking process ushers calcium into that cell. This can be problematic if it's a cancer cell and the unlocking signals the cell to divide.

One of the primary functions of a hormone is to stimulate cell proliferation (division). When a hormone unlocks that lock, it's like turning the ignition in a car and stepping on the gas pedal at the same time. That cell is revved up. You can see why this would be a bad thing to do with a cancer cell. And, unfortunately, many cancer cells have figured this out and rely on hormonally activated proliferation. The majority of breast cancers are developed from cells that are studded with estrogen receptors and utilize estrogen to drive their growth. The cells comprising many solid cancers have numerous insulin receptors on their surfaces and utilize insulin (a hormone) to drive growth. The pathway from the receptor to the DNA is often not an isolated one. In fact, most receptor-mediated growth pathways in cells interact with other pathways. For example, estrogen receptors cooperate with insulin receptors to epigenetically influence the DNA by uncoiling it. As you recall from our discussion on epigenetics, the genes that reside in the "relaxed" portions of DNA are transcribed, or "read" into certain proteins. In the case of estrogen and insulin, many of these proteins stimulate cell division and invasion. This is why estrogen is such a potent driver of cancer growth for cancer cells that are estrogen receptor–positive.

Cortisol is another example of a hormone that has significant impact on cancer risk. Cortisol is secreted as a part of our stress response. Chronic stress can chronically elevate cortisol, and this can have serious health implications. For example, increased cortisol results in an imbalanced immune response, which in turn increases IL-6 production. As we mentioned, IL-6 is an inflammatory cytokine that when elevated is associated with decreased survival in people with advanced cancer. High cortisol levels also result in decreased natural killer (NK) cell activity. In fact, severe life stress may cause an up to 50 percent reduction in NK cell activity by epigenetically preventing the transcription of genes in NK cells necessary for cellular activity. Reduction of NK cell activity leads to decreased immune surveillance against viral-infected cells and cancerous cells. The epigenetic effects of stress on the immune system are thus significant, as stress may increase our predisposition to autoimmune disease, infections, and cancer.

These are examples of why we focus on all five pathways. You can see that hormones intensely affect other pathways, such as inflammation and immunity, and we rely on the detoxification pathway to maintain hormonal homeostasis. This is true of all the pathways—they interact and rely on each other. The five pathways work in concert. When we are healthy, our life is a wonderful mel-

FIVE PATHWAY POINTS TO REMEMBER

We've identified one key point for each of the five pathways to help illustrate the power that is within us.

Immune

1. The human body contains trillions of specialized immune system cells that search for, identify, and destroy damaged cells, including cancer cells.

Inflammation

2. Prolonged inflammation creates tissue chaos, ultimately resulting in an environment that favors cancer development. The good news is that we can quench the inflammatory fires and heal the damage caused by chronic inflammation.

Hormones

3. Hormones are powerful messengers that often serve as growth signals for cells, which makes hormonal balance paramount to controlled cellular growth and cancer prevention.

Insulin Resistance

4. Cells are studded with insulin receptors and will use insulin to stimulate their proliferation, making insulin resistance a dangerous state that can, in fact, be reversed through diet and lifestyle.

Digestion/Detoxification

5. Our digestive/detoxification pathway provides us with critical nutrients and helps us to rid our system of toxic, cancer-causing substances.

ody, but when we are not well, we are out of tune and every off note impacts the entire orchestra's ability to perform.

The connection between the pathways continues further as we discuss insulin resistance. Insulin is actually a hormone that is secreted by the pancreas, an organ within the endocrine system. As we build our strong cancer prevention foundation, the insulin resistance pathway becomes a critical part of that platform.

4. INSULIN RESISTANCE

To understand the link between cancer prevention and insulin resistance, we must first take a closer look at sugar, glucose metabolism, and how insulin works. Let's start with glucose and work our way toward insulin and then insulin resistance.

The majority of dietary carbohydrates contain glucose. Sucrose (typically consumed as refined sugar but also present in fruit, some vegetables, and some seeds and nuts) and lactose (found in dairy products) contain glucose linked with one other sugar. Glucose in these sugars is easily absorbed. Most glucose in foods occurs in long-chained polysaccharides. Digestive enzymes, with the help of beneficial bacteria in our intestines, digest polysaccharides, allowing us to absorb glucose. Upon absorption, glucose is either immediately used to make energy, especially in brain cells and red blood cells, or it is shuttled across the cell membranes of liver cells, muscle cells, and fat cells by insulin. Inside these cells, the glucose is converted into its stored form, glycogen.

Our bodies rely on glucose to make energy. The pancreas releases two different hormones to meet the body's needs for glucose, while at the same time avoiding too much glucose in circulation. These hormones are insulin and glucagon. If you have decreased blood glucose levels, glucagon is secreted to stimulate the release of the stored glucose (glycogen) into the bloodstream. Glucagon also stimulates our liver cells to make glucose, a process called gluconeogenesis. On the other hand, if you have increased blood glucose levels, the pancreas secretes insulin. Insulin escorts glucose back into liver, muscle, and fat cells in order to decrease its levels in the blood. It is important to keep blood glucose levels within a normal range. If it drops too low, our cells won't have enough energy. However, if glucose levels are too high, the glucose creates damage to the blood vessels, which will, over time, lead to a number of health problems common to diabetics.

When we eat a diet that contains minimal refined sugar, exercise regularly, and have sufficient vitamin and mineral intake, blood sugar levels can be properly maintained. But if the diet has too many simple sugars and refined carbohydrates or if we skip meals, are under stress, and don't exercise, blood sugar levels will become elevated. The body manages this situation simply by increasing its production of insulin. The extra insulin matches the rise in blood sugar in order to efficiently transport the glucose into cells for storage and energy metabolism. However, over time, cells lose their ability to take in more glucose, a state characterized by insulin resistance. Essentially, cells shut their doors to glucose by preventing its chaperone, insulin, from entering. The "doors," or insulin receptors on an insulin-resistant cell, are altered so the insulin no longer fits into the receptor. With the loss of this fit, insulin cannot transport glucose across the cell membrane. Both the insulin and the glucose are left to circulate in the bloodstream.

Unfortunately, this strategy backfires, and the cells develop a strong need for the glucose that is barred from entering. In an effort to get glucose into cells, the pancreas secretes more insulin. Sadly, the receptors have not changed, and simply adding more insulin to the blood does not solve the problem. In fact, increased blood levels of insulin can create their own problems, particularly if there are cancer cells in the body. Simply put, insulin resistance feeds cancer.

How exactly does insulin resistance fuel cancer growth? Cancer cells have huge requirements for glucose because they have inefficient metabolism and require rapid growth to survive. Because of this, cancer cell membranes are loaded with insulin receptors. Even if some of the insulin receptors on cancer cells are resistant to glucose, there are so many insulin receptors that some will always be functional. This means when healthy cells are insulin resistant, cancer cells can still bind insulin and bring glucose into the cell. And it gets worse. In addition to escorting glucose across the cell membrane, when insulin binds to insulin receptors, several other intracellular pathways are activated, creating a waterfall of signals translated into the nucleus that tells the cell to grow and divide. Insulin has a helper in the form of insulin growth factor-1 (IGF-1). When insulin levels are elevated, so are IGF-1 levels; as the name implies, IGF-1 binds to insulin growth factor receptors and signals cellular proliferation. Some cancers rely almost exclusively on IGF-1 and insulin to stimulate their growth, and most cancers will utilize these molecules to spur their growth at least to some extent.

Because insulin resistance is such a strong driver of cancer growth, it is of paramount importance to break through this resistance. This is one reason we recommend eliminating dietary refined sugar and simple carbohydrates found in refined grains. Removing these insulin secretion triggers will lower blood insulin and IGF-1 levels. Regular exercise along with this diet adjustment supports healthy insulin receptors and is a powerful anti-cancer strategy. We'll discuss diet in a lot more detail in Chapter 5.

You may be wondering about fruit intake. After all, most fruits are high in sugar, and yet they are still considered healthful foods. Fruit does not need to be eliminated to address insulin resistance and cancer growth. That's because, in its whole form, most fruit is packed with fiber, vitamins, minerals, enzymes, and polyphenols, which are important antioxidant and anti-inflammatory molecules that give the fruit its vibrant color. This healthful combination of nutrients moderates the release of the fruit sugar, protects the blood vessels from potentially damaging effects of that sugar, and supports several other anti-proliferative, pro-repair and pro-apoptotic (cell death) effects in cancer cells. A study featured in the *Journal of Nutrition* demonstrated that having a smoothie containing whole blueberries twice a day for six weeks significantly improved insulin sensitivity in obese individuals. This doesn't surprise us, because blueberries are packed with potent flavonoids (the compounds that give them that bright blue color). Flavonoids have been shown to increase insulin sensitivity and lower blood sugar. These same flavonoids also stimulate the immune system and reduce inflammation. Add to this flavonoids' many other epigenetic influences on cancer cells and you begin to see why fruit and vegetables are such an important part of an anti-cancer plan. For instance, active compounds in fruit and vegetables free up DNA repair and tumor suppressor genes, allowing these genes to make repair proteins, proteins that slow cell division, and proteins that facilitate cell suicide if the damage is too great to be repaired.

Insulin resistance (also known as metabolic syndrome or syndrome X) is linked to more than cancer development. Insulin resistance can lead to diabetes and is a precursor to pancreatic failure. To reduce the risk of many illnesses, we must break the cycle of constant insulin secretion and allow the body to manage and maintain healthy blood sugar levels. The good news is that we can reverse insulin resistance. A combination of diet and lifestyle, specifically exercise, is the best way to do this. We'll discuss exercise in a lot more detail in Chapter 4.

Our fifth and final pathway is the digestion/detoxification pathway. While this may seem like two pathways, digestion and detoxification work so closely together and rely on each other so much that we treat them as one pathway.

5. DIGESTION/DETOXIFICATION

Virtually every function of the human body requires nutrients. Where do the organs, tissues, and cells of the body get their nutrition? From digesting the foods we eat. And how do we protect our cells, tissues, and organs from damage? With detoxification. Digestion and detoxification are the powerful one-two punch that both feeds our cells and protects them. Let's start with a quick look at digestion.

The digestive system begins in the mouth and ends with the anus. There is a lot of activity that goes on between those two points after you ingest food. Starting with the saliva in your mouth, and including stomach acid, bile secreted from the gall bladder, pancreatic enzymes from the pancreas, and intestinal enzymes, food doesn't stand much of a chance in the digestive tract. Food is mechanically and chemically broken down so the nutrients can be absorbed through the intestines while the food byproducts are eliminated. It's also in the intestines where our immune cells, in concert with beneficial bacteria, sample food for disease-causing bacteria and other contaminants. Immune cells in the intestines? Absolutely. In fact, about 70 percent of our immune cells live in the digestion pathway. These immune cells serve a critical function as an immune barrier to the disease-causing microorganisms in our food. When our digestive system is healthy, so too is our immune system. Once again, you can see how the pathways are so intimately connected.

Healthy intestinal absorption is critical to get the nutrients we need while minimizing the absorption of harmful substances. Unfortunately, sometimes the lining of the intestines can become too permeable, allowing toxic particles to pass through the lining into the bloodstream, which can overwhelm the liver's capacity to detoxify these compounds.

When the intestinal lining becomes too permeable, it's called leaky gut syndrome. Think of it like a food colander with holes that are too large. Using such a colander could cause the grapes you are washing to slip through and go right down the drain. What causes those "holes" to develop in our intestinal lining? There are several factors:

- Bacterial overgrowth (see sidebar about bacteria on page 30)
- Inadequate digestion in the stomach
- Inflammatory intolerance of specific foods
- Free radical damage
- Certain medications, such as antibiotics

The good news is that the advice in the coming chapters will help you avoid and even reverse leaky gut syndrome.

Optimal digestion and detoxification require a healthy liver. The liver is really "command central" when it comes to detoxification. In addition to breaking down harmful substances, the liver also activates and stores nutrients that can be used later. The liver works hard for us 24/7.

Compounds absorbed from the digestive tract are immediately taken to the liver. The liver serves a key detoxifying and protective role by screening these compounds for any that might cause cellular damage. Through the activity of hundreds of detoxification enzymes, the liver turns toxic compounds into harmless waste. These same enzymes are dual purpose because, in addition to detoxifying toxins, they can also convert compounds into useful forms that the body can actually use. This is how we activate many of the vitamins, antioxidants, fats, and other nutrients contained in food into bioactive compounds that are used by our cells.

The liver produces about 100 different enzymes and proteins that carry out the complex process of detoxification. The enzymes are collectively known as cytochrome P450 (cP450), and the proteins are conjugating compounds. Detoxification consists of a two-step process to render toxins harmless, and if there is a problem with either of these two processes, reactive molecules that are toxic to cells and their DNA will be released into the body. These toxins are considered carcinogenic, or cancer causing, because they can damage DNA. It is thus very important that both phases of liver detoxification are working optimally.

Phase I of the detoxification process converts the compound into a water-soluble toxic intermediate. Phase II utilizes different proteins to bind to the toxic intermediates turning them into non-reactive, water-soluble, non-toxic compound that can be excreted in urine or stool. Health problems can occur if:

- either system becomes impaired,

- there is an increase in exposure to environmental toxins,

- we eat a poor diet that is deficient in the nutrients required by cP450 enzymes to function, or

- we have an overgrowth of harmful intestinal bacteria that contributes to leaky gut and a subsequent influx of toxic compounds.

Any one of these factors can put undue stress on the detoxification pathway, causing a buildup of cancer-causing toxic compounds.

Balanced detoxification activity is critical. When there is an imbalance with the detoxification phases, the result can be incomplete detoxification and cell damage. Underactive cP450 enzymes will not effectively break down dietary and environmental toxins. On the other hand, it is also problematic if the activity of the cP450 enzymes outpaces the supply of phase II conjugating compounds, since the intermediary toxins are often more reactive and DNA-damaging than their parent compounds.

Epigenetic factors that decrease cP450 genetic transcription and therefore activity include:

- Nutritional deficiencies, including protein deficiency
- Fasting
- High carbohydrate diet
- Grapefruit juice (specifically harigenin found in grapefruit juice)
- Vitamin A or C deficiency
- Bacterial toxins
- The aging process
- Some medications (benzodiazepines, antihistamines, and cimetidine)

Conversely, epigenetic factors that can increase the genetic transcription and therefore activity of cP450 enzymes include:

- Alcohol intake
- Smoking (including second-hand smoke)
- Some medications (acetaminophen and anti-seizure medications)
- Iron deficiency
- A high-protein diet
- Hydrocarbons formed during charcoal grilling

The advice provided in the following chapters will help support proper balance among the two phases of detoxification. In addition, there are liver detoxification tests available that measure phase I and phase II activity. These tests must be ordered by a licensed healthcare professional. As you can see, supporting and enhancing the digestion/detoxification pathway becomes a critical component to our cancer prevention plan.

WHAT'S NEXT?

Now that you have met the pathways and have a pretty solid understanding of how they work on their own and together, it's important to know how to support them. The health of these pathways determines the health of your internal landscape. The coming chapters will provide you with practical strategies you can incorporate into your daily routine. These strategies will maximize your opportunity to prevent cancer and to live life with vitality. It's time to thrive, and we'll show you how!

 **HIGH FIVE TIP** *Be open to change. Mahatma Gandhi inspired people when he said "You must be the change you want to see in the world." This is true of the world that is you. To embrace change is to embrace knowledge. Just by making it this far in the book demonstrates that you are open to the information that will enhance your knowledge to become the change you want to see. Stay the course and be open to change!*

CHAPTER

MORE **LOVE, LAUGHTER,** AND **JOY** PLEASE!

fter our presentation in Seattle, an elderly gentleman came up to us and said with obvious surprise in his voice "That was a very interesting talk." He continued, "Honestly, I sat in the back because I thought I might doze off a bit, which is what I typically do at these things." We laughed and almost in unison we asked, "Why did you come?" He smiled a big smile and pointed across the room at a woman talking to another woman and said, "That's my wife. We've been married for nearly 30 years." He proudly continued, "She had breast cancer more than five years ago, and she just loves coming to these things so I always go with her."

That's love! Even though he anticipated taking an hour-long nap in a room full of strangers, he came anyway to support his wife. And when he said, "That's my wife" he stood a little taller and his chest broadened with loving pride. You could feel their connection even though they were on opposite sides of the room. It felt good, even to those of us merely witnessing it. Mother Teresa once said "Do not think that love in order to be genuine has to be extraordinary." Rather the contrary is often true: A simple gesture, like sitting through a boring lecture (which, of course, ours are not!), is a small price to pay to show the one you love that she is supported and admired. What you will discover in this chapter is that love, laughter, and feeling joy actually have physiological effects on your internal landscape. That's right, these feelings and actions can help to epigenetically influence your cells in a positive way!

It may seem odd to begin the Five to Thrive plan with "love, laughter, and joy." Perhaps you were expecting us to kick things off with diet or exercise or even dietary supplements—a concrete sub-

FIVE SIMPLE THINGS YOU CAN DO TO ADD MORE LOVE TO YOUR LIFE

1. Encourage Gratitude

Being grateful for others fills your heart with appreciation. You can encourage gratitude in your life by starting your day with thoughts of gratefulness. Before you even get out of bed, think of at least one thing, situation, or being (human or animal) you are grateful for. Let yourself appreciate this object of gratitude for a few moments. You could also keep a gratitude journal and, each night before bed, jot down the things you were grateful for that day.

2. Love Meditation

Think about several times when you felt loved and picture those times in your mind's eye. These are now your love meditations. Take some time each week to listen to relaxing music and think about the love meditations you have created. Recall how you felt, whom you were with, and how appreciated and loved you felt at that time. When you are done, take some full, deep breaths and let those moments sink into the very fabric of your being.

3. Speak From the Heart

This week, tell someone you love either verbally or in writing why you love them and why you appreciate their love. It doesn't have to be a big, drawn out event—just a simple act of you speaking the truth and reminding yourself and others that you experience love and are grateful for the opportunity to share it. Be authentic in your expression.

4. Favorite Past Times

What are your top three things you just love to do? Keep track of how much time you spend each week doing one or more of those three things. Relish the moments you do get to enjoy them, and if you can, give each of these loved activities even a few more minutes of your time each week.

5. Love Yourself

Take time to appreciate something about yourself. Maybe it's a characteristic or attribute. Or maybe it's a special talent. With a smile on your face, give yourself a hug or a pat on the back. We all have gifts to share, and it's important that we recognize and love the gifts that we carry.

ject you can really sink your teeth into. While all of these are also important, we wanted to begin with love because we firmly believe that only when you support your health from a place of love, will you find success. It makes sense that if we begin from a place of self-loathing or fear, negativity and emptiness will be reinforced. Good athletes figured this out long ago. If a tennis player laments every bad shot and tells herself before each shot, "Don't take your eyes off the ball," she will likely take her eyes off the ball. If, instead, she counsels herself to keep her eyes on the ball, she is more likely to have the solid shot she is anticipating.

Physical health that is sustainable must begin in a positive place, a place inspired by love of life, love of yourself, and love of others. But this can be difficult when we are paralyzed by fear of cancer. For those of us who have seen firsthand what cancer can do, we understand the fear that accompanies it. Cancer is one of the most feared diseases of all time. This is not altogether unreasonable. Cancer is a scary illness, and its treatments are often more frightening than the disease. On one level, this fear is a healthy response to a terrifying situation. Our fear is an expression of our desire to live. We are afraid of the cancer and its treatments, because we love living our lives. If we can tap into that part of our fear, then being afraid can actually guide us back to our place of strength. If we just focus on the fear itself, we can forget why we are truly afraid and become lost and paralyzed in the fear. The love that spawns our fear is its antidote. To understand how love can heal us from the fear, we must first understand the physical ramifications associated with our fears. Power comes in knowing, so let's get to know a little bit more about fear, as well as the anxiety and stress associated with our fears.

FEAR FACTOR

For those of you who are living in the United States, we would venture a guess that you can quickly remember where you were and what you were doing when you first heard about the 9/11 terrorist attacks in New York City, Washington, DC, and over Pennsylvania. Many of us witnessed the horror on TV and we were paralyzed by the sight of the Twin Towers collapse. The stress and anxiety caused by that fearful event was heart-wrenching. We were afraid for the people at the sites of the attacks, afraid for our country, and afraid for our loved ones and ourselves. But what you may not realize is that even for those of us who merely witnessed the event on television, that experience likely had a long-lasting physiological effect on our bodies.

A 2008 paper in the *Archives of General Psychiatry* found that randomly selected people who reported significant stress and anxiety after the 9/11 terrorist attacks had higher rates of heart disease up to three years later. Interestingly, nearly all of the people in the study had only seen the attacks on TV.

This example illustrates that stress, anxiety, and fear can have very real and long-lasting physical consequences. We know that chronic stress (and therefore the fears associated with that stress) can

- weaken immunity, specifically immune cell activation;
- release an excess of inflammatory hormones;
- deplete vitamins and minerals required by our stress response;
- disrupt the movement and integrity of our intestines and compromise digestion; and
- elevate blood sugar levels and accelerate tissue damage from this excessive sugar.

The stress response, which has been hardwired to keep us safe from harm, can actually do the opposite. When our stress response is chronic, it begins to unravel the function of each of our key bodily pathways. At the same time, long lasting stress can inhibit DNA repair and turn on cell-growth pathways. The combined effects pillage our internal landscape, leaving us exposed and vulnerable to diseases such as heart disease and cancer.

While acute stress, like acute fear, can be a life-saving response to imminent danger, sustained stress can drown us. The body's internal stress response was designed to help us fight danger or run for our lives and is aptly named the "fight or flight" response. When we feel threatened or under stress, stress hormones (adrena-

FIVE GUIDELINES ABOUT LOVE, LAUGHTER, AND JOY

1. SEEK OUT SOCIAL SUPPORT. Don't underestimate the dangers of isolation. If you don't have a strong support system with family and friends, consider joining a group like a book club, taking a class, or volunteering.

2. YOU CAN CULTIVATE LAUGHTER. Watch funny movies, hang out with funny friends, start laughing even if nothing is funny, and do whatever it takes to laugh frequently. The comedian Milton Berle once said, "Laughter is an instant vacation." Take an instant vacation today!

3. HAVE AN APPRECIATIVE ATTITUDE. Some researchers have found that gratitude can improve our sense of happiness more than we might realize. Remember, gratitude is a feeling that yearns for expression.

4. BE OPEN TO OPTIMISM. Is the glass half full or half empty? Work at being positive right now, in this moment,. The optimism that you experience today will bring you a great day tomorrow because tomorrow is a gift and you get to open it!

5. GET REAL. Being real means being authentic with yourself and with others. Authentic behavior helps create trust, support, and true joy. Be yourself and nurture the courage to express your feelings. Make sure your feelings, actions, and words match up.

line, noradrenaline also called norepinephrine, and cortisol) are released within seconds of the perceived threat. These hormones surge throughout the body and activate several other chemicals to help us cope with the situation.

Inflammatory compounds such as nuclear factor kappa-beta (NF-kB); interleukins such as IL-6, IL-1, IL-12, and IL-8; C-reactive protein (CRP); and homocysteine are released. These compounds activate several processes, such as the release of stored glucose and amino acids, which are quickly used to make energy. Heart rate, blood pressure, blood volume, lung strength, and eye pupil dilation are all increased to facilitate our capacity to make a quick escape or fight the threat. Within minutes, blood flow increases throughout the body and increases cellular growth and proliferation. This is all supremely helpful if we sustain an acute injury or if we are confronted by an acute threat, such as a mugger on a darkened street. But what happens when this threat is constant—when there's not a mugger chasing us, but rather constant daily deadlines or—worse yet—the constant threat of cancer hanging over our heads?

In a prolonged state of stress the continuous release of stress hormones, instead of protecting us, begins to unravel our internal homeostasis. The hormones released under stress keep our bodies functioning as if they were repairing a wound or responding to imminent danger all the time. The blood pounding adrenaline surge, instead of receding, remains. Over months and years, it wreaks havoc on what are normally exquisitely choreographed cellular processes. The beautiful cellular dance is replaced with chaotic, disorderly, and unregulated cellular activities. The function of our organs, tissues, and cells begins to deteriorate, and chronic disease enters the scene. In addition to increasing the risk of cancer, chronic stress puts us at risk for developing infections, ulcers, heart disease, digestive issues, and mental illness.

When you are afraid and running from a mugger, the ensuing stress response is very effective at assisting your escape. But when you are constantly afraid of being attacked by cancer, your continued stress response may actually help facilitate the very thing you fear: cancer.

Obviously, it's not as simple as just recognizing you are afraid and saying, "I'm not afraid anymore!" The practical advice found in this chapter and the chapters to follow will give you a comprehensive strategy to help you feel more empowered and less fearful. Successfully overcoming fear and its physical effects requires a multipronged approach. In addition to investigating the source and reasons for our fears and establishing a psychological strategy to dismantle them, there are several other aspects that need support. For example, a low glycemic, whole foods–based diet will help control blood sugar ups and downs that otherwise can cause anxiety and even panic. Regular exercise releases "feel-good" hormones (endorphins) that can help reduce feelings of fear and anxiety. Certain dietary supplements, such as L-theanine (brand name Suntheanine®), L-glycine, 5-hydroxytryptophan, and herbal extracts of ashwaganda (*Withania somnifera*) or valerian (*Valeriana officinalis*), can help ease anxiety. There are many ways to conquer fear and positively influence your wellbeing even on a cellular level.

Remember, it doesn't pay to fret about the future. In fact, the only place fear can exist is in the future where we can only *imagine* what may happen. When we stay focused on the present, we leave no room for fear. One way to stay focused on the here and now is to be in tune with our actions, reactions, and the actions of others—especially the act of loving.

Love can either be a noun, love for someone, or a verb, to feel love. To feel love requires attention and action. Just as you would learn a foreign language if you took up residence in a different country, you can learn the language of love to live in a world without chronic fear. To begin the process, lets dissect what it takes to experience happiness, the catalyst for love.

THE SCIENCE OF HAPPINESS

Were you born to be happy or unhappy? It was previously thought that our ability to be happy was genetic. We were either hardwired for happiness or destined for doom. Not so! In fact, a movement called "positive psychology" has recently emerged. This new field studies the health effects of positive emotions and life satisfaction and how they can be encouraged in patients.

What does the "science of happiness" show us so far? People who are happier tend to be healthier and live longer. Paul J. Hershberger, PhD, refers to several studies in his article featured in the October 2005 edition of the journal *Family Medicine*. For example, he evaluated the emotional content of the handwritten biographies of 180 Catholic nuns and found that the nuns who wrote more positively lived significantly longer. At the end of his literature review Hershberger concluded: "Happy people have better quality of life, and research in the behavioral, social, and medical sciences is continuing to identify other benefits of happiness, including better health."

Happy people don't just find themselves in this state of mind. People who are generally happy create their own happiness. Studies show that happy people have more of a tendency to do these five things:

1. Express gratitude on a regular basis

2. Be more consistently optimistic

3. Engage in frequent acts of kindness

4. Appreciate joyful events

5. Practice forgiveness

Sometimes it helps to look at happiness through the eyes of a child. A child's optimism, even when tested by time-outs, long car rides, or eating peas, lies at the ready and erupts in full force as soon as the last ghastly pea is swallowed. There is nothing quite like watching a child laugh and clap with excitement and joy. Observe children at play and you will likely witness the masterful enactment of these tenets of happiness. And then ask yourself, "How can I do more of these five things in my life?"

Some preliminary research shows that doing something very simple like recognizing good things can increase gratitude and is associated with greater happiness and less depression. In one study, participants were asked to write down every night three positive things that happened during the day. They also wrote down why they felt the good things happened. This journaling activity lasted for one week. The anti-depression benefits of this simple

EMBRACING THE HEALING PHILOSOPHY OF YOGA

There is a Hindu greeting that is just one simple word: *Namaste*. But that simple greeting packs a great deal of meaning: "I honor the place in you in which the entire universe dwells, I honor the place in you that is of love, integrity, wisdom, and peace. When you are in that place in you, and I am in that place in me, we are one."

As you continue on your joyful cancer prevention path, we share with you this simple love-filled greeting: **Namaste.**

activity lasted for three months. This is an example of something we can all do. Even if we only do this every now and then, the benefits will be ongoing.

Let's look at an example that may hit closer to home—optimism and ovarian cancer. A 2006 published study in *Psychosomatic Medicine* demonstrated that women with ovarian cancer undergoing chemotherapy who were more optimistic (specifically "dispositional optimism" which is feeling good about the future), had lower levels of distress, higher levels of perceived quality of life, and a greater decline in the CA-125 tumor marker test. CA-125 is a tumor marker produced by ovarian cancer cells and other inflamed cells that shed into the blood. Measurements of CA-125 are used to assess the activity of ovarian cancer, and treatment success is measured, in part, by its ability to decrease CA-125. This study demonstrated that optimism impeded ovarian cancer growth.

Social isolation and feeling unloved can be a detriment to good health and happiness. A 2005 study looking at women with advanced ovarian cancer found that the women who felt a sense of closeness and intimacy with a loved one (what the researchers called social attachment) had lower levels of IL-6. IL-6 is an inflammatory marker associated with cancer growth. Research has also shown than people with certain advanced cancers (ovarian, breast, prostate, and others) who have elevated IL-6 levels have a poorer prognosis. The bottom line: social support and feeling loved can reduce internal inflammation and decrease cancer growth.

Another interesting study from 2006, published in *Brain, Behavior, and Immunity,* found that people receiving the flu vaccine who felt they were in a positive marital relationship had a higher antibody response (meaning the vaccine was more effective) than those who had lower marital satisfaction. The researchers concluded that there is importance in evaluating the relationship between psychosocial factors and immunity. In fact, immunity is heavily influenced by emotions and vice versa. Many of the molecules, namely cytokines and interleukins, that activate our immune responses are the same molecules that create emotions generated in the brain. To make this even more interesting, these same molecules influence the activity of our digestion. In essence, our thoughts, feelings, and bodily functions influence each other through a shared molecular language. Candace Pert, PhD, a renowned scientist, coined this currency in the title of her landmark book, *Molecules of Emotion: The Science Behind Mind-Body Medicine* (Simon & Schuster, 1999). The modern field of psychoneuroimmunology is devoted to studying this interplay and has given rise to the concept that our immune system is absolutely interconnected with our emotional and cognitive processes.

Keeping our immunity strong may require that we give way to expressing the full range of our emotions. While the ultimate goal is to experience love, by way of experiencing happiness and optimism while banishing chronic fear, it is also important to make room for emotions such as sadness. "Happiness is not the absence of sadness," says David Spiegel, MD, medical director of the Center for Integrative Medicine at Stanford University School of Medicine. "Phony happiness is not good," he concludes; we concur.

People who consistently suppress sad emotions are basically teaching themselves to suppress other emotions as well, including happiness. According to Spiegel, people who suppress emotions have more of a tendency to become depressed or anxious. If sadness is your most genuine reaction to life events, then expressing this grief is the best way to interact with life—in other words, to be fully alive and present. While emotions are by their very nature temporary, they all deserve to see the light of day. That means that one of the keys to happiness is to not only express yourself but also be yourself.

Expressing yourself is living life with authenticity. Being authentic is being consistent with your thoughts, feelings, words, and actions. It means you are congruent with what you say and what you do and that you believe in both your words and your actions. If you sense that someone is being inauthentic, what are the feelings that arise? Perhaps it makes you feel untrusting or you immediately discount the message and the messenger. In the business world, there is a big push for "authentic leadership." The reason is simple: authenticity builds trust and openness and helps people feel more comfortable.

Authentic living can be a rare find. So many of us are trying to live in ways that are not consistent with who we really are. Many

A CASE OF RESILIENCE *By Dr. Alschuler*

I have a dear friend who is 71 years old, as spunky as they come, and the picture of good health. She is intensely inquisitive of everyone who has the good fortune of meeting her. With focused determination, in a matter of minutes, she can extract the most intimate details even from the most reticent person. At the same time, she has a constant twinkle in her eye and a belly laugh ready to erupt at any moment. Around a table filled with her friends, she is often the center of lively conversation. At one of these dinner gatherings a while ago, I asked her, "What do you most attribute your good health to?" She laughed, "My good health is most certainly the result of my ability to survive my bad habits." Perhaps she was referring to her evening bourbon cocktail or her disdain for structured exercise routines. She does have a few bad habits to be sure, but as the evening progressed, I wasn't thinking of those. I watched her listen to her friends with complete compassion while gently and persistently pointing out the silver lining in every cloud, and simply delighting in the joy of being with people she loves. I thought about her past too, and the deep adversity and loss she has experienced. It then dawned on me that the real secret to her health and vitality was resilience — her unceasing ability to rebound from all manner of disappointments and to emerge into a confident embrace of life within and around her. Her resilience seeps into those she interacts with as she buoys them up, praises them, and revels in their unique brilliance. You cannot help but feel better after an interaction with her. She lives life with this expectation: She will swing at anything that life throws her way, she will make contact, and she will take pleasure in wherever the ball flies. I smile as I think of her as she ends her day, likely snuggled in her bed watching one of her favorite TV shows, eager to fall asleep so that she can start another day tomorrow!

of us try to live up to unrealistic expectations, and sometimes even if these expectations are not our own. This leads squarely into a life of incongruence. Living or acting in a way that is "normal" but inconsistent with what we truly believe is the foundation for an inauthentic life. Going through the motions of relationships, work, and activities without our hearts fully engaged is living life on "auto pilot" and can be a lonely, unfulfilling path.

You can develop and practice authenticity by enlisting some help. Call on someone close to you to be your authentic witness and to inform you when she/he senses you are not being "real". Choose someone you trust who will be tactful and gentle. Also, at the end of the day think of times throughout the day when you may have been inauthentic. What would you have done or said differently to have been more authentic? Finally, as you consider your life, find the courage to ask yourself what parts of your life are simply just not you. What changes could you make to bring you—all of you— fully into your life? Many people who have had cancer describe the diagnosis as their "wake-up call." By staring at their own mortality, they are given the opportunity to confront the meaning of their life. Many of these people make significant changes based on their diagnosis. They may change jobs, relationships, their lifestyle—all of which are changes toward living their lives with authenticity. The key is to not wait for a cancer diagnosis to make this transformation.

BIG BELLY LAUGH

We have a good friend and colleague, Jacob Schor, ND, who, as a naturopathic oncologist, believes that laughter is the best medicine. He has written articles on the subject and has even lectured to other healthcare professionals as to how they can incorporate laughter into their treatment protocols and patient visits. Why is he so adamant? As Jacob says, you can't argue with the scientific literature, folks!

In 2010 Schor did a literature review on laughter that was published in the *Natural Medicine Journal* (www.naturalmedicinejournal.com). Schor looked at studies involving the effects of laughter on allergic asthma, skin conditions, anxiety, depression, and even the immune system. His conclusion? "The scientific literature demonstrates that the effects of humor and laughter on health are far-ranging and numerous."

Perhaps the most fascinating aspect of laughter for us is the fact that it impacts us on a cellular level—it can epigenetically influence how our cells behave. Just the simple act of experiencing a big belly laugh can turn on certain genes and turn off other genes.

Japanese researchers found that laughter improves immune function and blood glucose levels by modulating natural killer (NK) activity in diabetic patients. What was the research method? Funny videos. In one of their studies, they recruited people who were attending a diabetes management seminar. One day they watched funny videos and the other day they attended the educational seminar. Amazingly, just laughing at the comical videos up-regulated at least 27 genes that increase NK activity, and this effect lasted for four hours after the video was over.

Specific to cancer, a 2005 literature review featured in the *Clinical Journal of Oncology Nursing* summarized studies on laughter and immunity in people diagnosed with cancer and found that laughter stimulated a positive immune response, helped control pain and anxiety, and promoted general wellness. Based on their review of the scientific literature, the authors concluded, "Humor can be an effective intervention that impacts the health and well-being of patients with cancer."

Surprisingly, even the act of laughing, even if you are not laughing at anything funny, improves mood and health. This has led to a new form of therapy called laughter therapy, which utilizes laughter as a therapeutic intervention. Laughter therapy has been studied in a variety of settings and has demonstrated positive effects on depression, insomnia, and sleep quality in people with depression, people diagnosed with cancer, the elderly, and others. The key is to find ways to laugh.

Famous American poet and essayist E. E. Cummings once wrote, "The most wasted of all days is one without laughter." Life is precious—don't waste any more days.

JOY TO YOU AND ME

Wouldn't it be great if there were a system in the brain that helped us feel more joy? There is! It's called the mesolimbic pathway. Simply speaking, this is the part of the brain that is associated with the feeling of joy. More technically speaking, it's the brain's system that links certain behaviors with feelings of reward and reinforces those feelings through the emotions of pleasure and happiness. This circuit relies on the release of dopamine, a neurotransmitter that serves many functions, including stimulation of positive feelings.

The mesolimbic pathway has instant and long-lasting effects. If we touch a hot plate, for example, in an instant the nerves in our hands communicate with our brain and we immediately drop the plate. The same is true when humans experience joy. As a child swings on a swing set, his smile and laughter is associated with the release of chemicals that tells his brain that he is having fun and experiencing joy. When the child later walks through the park and sees the swing set, he will in an instant run to jump on the swing; he is joyful simply anticipating the upcoming swinging.

The human body is filled with complex pathways, chemical releases, and internal structures to keep us healthy and vibrant. It's good to know that there are even physiological systems in place to help us be more joyful. How do we maximize the potential of our mesolimbic pathway? We take advantage of its consistent programming for positive reinforcement.

If we are trying to train a puppy, we will reward good behavior, most likely with a yummy treat. The way we reinforce feelings of joyfulness is to reward the behaviors by doing them frequently. If you find joy in gardening, schedule an appointment with the garden each week or more! If you enjoy reading, carve out some time each day to read, even if it's just a few pages at night. Frequency of joyful activities will help reinforce joy in your life.

Unfortunately, because the mesolimic pathway relies on rewards to reinforce it, it can also be influenced by unhealthy behaviors such as smoking or alcohol use. If we find pleasure after smoking, that behavior will be reinforced and we will desire another cigarette. Rewiring that behavior to overcome the addiction can be very difficult. An important part of removing unhealthy habits is to substitute enjoyable, healthier activities for the unhealthy ones. Remember, to be successful, these substituted healthy habits also need to make you feel happy.

The idea is to utilize healthy activities as a way to hardwire our mesolimbic pathway. By repeating joyous activities or finding joy in healthy habits, we can more easily train our brain to want to do those activities regularly.

Take a moment to identify five healthy activities that bring you joy. Congratulations! You've just identified a new focus for your mesolimbic pathway plan. It can be that easy. Reinforcing these five areas of focus through repetition will strengthen your feeling of happiness. Out of this happiness, you will experience a greater capacity for love. Out of love, you will find a source of continuous inspiration to live your life with happiness, authenticity, humor, and vibrant health.

We began this chapter with an inspiring quote from Mother Teresa and we will end with one as well: "A joyful heart is the inevitable result of a heart burning with love."

Love, laughter, and joy—in the race against cancer, this is the trifecta!

 **HIGH FIVE TIP** *Take time in each day to focus on others—how you feel about others and how you interact with them. One of our favorite quotes from famed poet Maya Angelou is "I've learned that people will forget what you said, people will forget what you did, but people will never forget how you made them feel." How can you make someone you care about feel special today? One of the most powerful ways to experience love is to give it away freely and authentically.*

CHAPTER 4

WE ARE **MEANT** TO **MOVE**

"I know I should exercise more," a woman tells us after one of our presentations. "But, you know, I'm just not the spandex type. Staying fit was never an issue for me so I didn't really have to exercise. But now that I'm in my 40s, everything has changed." It was pretty obvious that she was frustrated. And she was stuck with only one vision of exercise. Although we love what Jane Fonda and the 80s exercise movement did to promote physical activity, the hangover of that stereotype lingers. Many people have one view of exercise—tight-fitting clothes, mirrored rooms, and sweating on aerobic mats or weight machines alongside body builders. In this chapter we will deconstruct stereotypes about exercise and help you look at fitness through a new lens. In fact, let's not even call it exercise. Let's simply think of it as *movement*.

Our bodies "talk" to us. If we sit for too long, lift a heavy object, or try out a new exercise, our bodies may speak the language of stiffness, achiness, or even pain. Yes, some movements can be uncomfortable, but the reality is that movement equals freedom; we are truly meant to move.

Let's break this down into simple terms. In order for anything to be able to move, it requires the following:

1. Rigid bar = our bones
2. Fulcrum or hinge point = our joints
3. Weight that is moved = our body
4. Force or mechanical energy = our muscles

These required parts work in proportion to each other. If the weight becomes too heavy to be "moved," the bones become too weak, the joints too stiff from disuse or disrepair, or the muscles too weak from inactivity, we will begin to lose vital mechanical energy. With the loss of this energy, we further compromise our ability to move, and we enter a vicious cycle of becoming sedentary for long periods of time. Henry Ford was quoted as saying, "Money is like an arm or a leg—use it or lose it." Just like using your money, you can use movement as an investment in your health. This chapter will show you how to earn big dividends so your health can prosper in the future.

Before we dig into the various ways to be physical, let's take a quick look at why activity is so important.

EPIGENETICS AND EXERCISE

We'll discuss epigenetics and exercise, but first a little physics. Sir Isaac Newton, commonly known as the father of physics, established several fundamental laws that govern motion. Newton's first law taught us that there is a natural tendency for an object to keep doing what it is doing. This law can be applied to us. If we are active, we will keep being active. If we are sedentary, we will remain so. This is Newton's law of inertia.

Newton's second law, is that the heavier the object, the more force is required to move it. This is why it can be more difficult and take extra effort to be physically active if we carry extra weight.

Finally, Newton also showed us that for every action there is a reaction. Remember those clicking balls suspended by strings that people used to keep on their desks or coffee tables? Allow one ball to hit its neighbor, and all the balls will continue moving by transferring their momentum into each other through their collisions. Those clicking balls are called Newton's cradle. And it's this third law of motion that leads us to epigentics and exercise. Now let's see how Newton's laws of motion help us understand the epigenetic impact of exercise on cancer prevention.

For every action we take, there is a reaction inside our bodies. It's also true that lack of action leads to inertia. After all, if we don't move that first ball, all the balls will remain still. Let's translate this

EXERCISING IN A SMALL TOWN

By Dr. Alschuler

Mary (not her real name) was a patient of mine who was concerned about cancer. She had never been diagnosed with cancer, but both of her parents and one of her sisters had died of cancer so she was worried. Mary wanted to do whatever she could to decrease her risk. It turned out the main thing missing in Mary's health plan was exercise. She was not physically active at all.

Mary decided she would begin a daily walking regimen. To motivate herself, she signed up for a fundraising walk that was to take place nine months from the time she started walking. Mary lived in a small town and owned a store in the town's center. She knew most of the people in the town, so when she started her daily walking routine, everyone in town noticed. After several months, Mary started to feel—and look—healthier. Despite challenges the economy presented to her business, she felt more optimistic than she had in years. Her optimism spilled over into her interactions with her customers and her neighbors. Several months into her new walking routine, some neighbors approached Mary and asked if they could join her.

By the time the fundraising walk came around, Mary signed up a dozen people to participate with her. Mary not only moved her own body, she also moved her community into greater health.

into the clicking balls of health inside our bodies that get put into motion when we are physically active.

The key to physical activity is oxygen. Simply stated, being physically active gives us the breath of life. As we move, blood vessels throughout the body dilate in order to increase the flow of oxygen to our working muscles, lungs, and heart. The more we exercise, the more conditioned we become. A big part of this conditioning is the increased efficiency of getting oxygen to our muscles. Another key component of conditioning is increased efficiency of our muscles' ability to utilize oxygen to make energy which powers continued movement. That's why people who are physically fit are not panting and out of breath after a brisk walk like their unfit counterparts.

Energy is not only a requisite for movement, it is also required for every process conducted within our cells, tissues, and organs. Therefore because movement oxygenates our body, it supports the activity in all of our cells. This is one of the reasons people who are regularly active tend to have more energy. On the other hand, when we are lacking sufficient oxygen, our cells behave in much the same way as we behave if we are out of breath. Think about it—we gasp, become light-headed, perhaps dizzy, and maybe even faint when we can't get enough oxygen. Our cells need a constant supply of oxygen in order to carry out the numerous metabolic processes necessary to keep us alive. Without it, our cells begin to act "dizzy." Key cellular functions become compromised, and cells become inefficient. If cells are deprived of oxygen for too long, they will eventually self-destruct.

Cells receive oxygen at the same time waste products of metabolism are being removed—oxygen in, carbon dioxide out. So another consequence of lack of oxygen is the accumulation of toxic waste products inside the cell. Eventually this toxic overload causes cells to become weak and damaged. Cells in virtually every nook and cranny of our body, in every major system, and in every key pathway must remove their waste products in exchange for the required oxygen in order to function properly.

The benefits of movement are far-reaching. We don't believe in magic bullets, but we feel movement is as close as you can get. Remember, one of the ways we prioritize diet, lifestyle activities, and dietary supplements is based on how many pathways are positively epigenetically influenced. In the case of exercise, *all* five pathways are significantly enhanced:

- *Immune system.* Regular exercise increases the activity of natural killer cells (NK cells) and cytotoxic T cells (CD8 cells), both of which are critical immune weapons used to destroy cancer. In one clinical study involving 53 postmenopausal breast cancer survivors, those who were assigned to the exercise group (using a stationary bike three times per week for 15 weeks) had significant increases in the cytotoxic activity of their NK cells compared to the non-exercising control group.

- **Inflammatory response.** Regular exercise is associated with lowered levels of several key blood-borne markers of chronic inflammation, namely high sensitivity C-reactive protein (hs-CRP) and homocysteine. In a 16-week clinical trial with 63 sedentary individuals (65–95 years old), 45 minutes of aerobic exercise three times per week plus strength training using resistance bands three times weekly resulted in a 26 percent reduction of hs-CRP.

- **Hormonal balance.** While exercise is associated with a transient increase in stress hormones, such as cortisol, regular exercise improves the sensitivity of the feedback loops that regulate the production of stress hormones. This increases our adaptability to stress and helps prevent abnormal stress-induced cortisol secretion. And exercise influences more than stress hormones. A 2010 study featured in *Obstetrics and Gynecology International* showed that exercise helped ease menopausal symptoms in postmenopausal women. As an added benefit, the women reported improvements in psychological health and overall quality of life.

- **Insulin resistance.** Exercise can actually *reverse* insulin resistance. Some research indicates that exercise is also the most potent strategy for preventing insulin resistance. Exercise is particularly effective at reducing insulin resistance in older adults. Clinical studies have demonstrated significant improvements in sugar metabolism with aerobic and/or resistance exercise training in middle-aged and older men and women. Exercise reduces fat content of muscles, improves tone of skeletal muscle, and increases blood flow, all of which decrease insulin resistance.

- **Digestion/detoxification.** Regular exercise improves all aspects of digestive function and is particularly effective at relieving constipation. Exercise also stimulates liver detoxification. Exercise's impact on the detoxification pathway is one of the reasons it is so important in cancer prevention. Regular exercise will increase the inactivation of carcinogens (cancer-causing chemicals), specifically by enhancing our most important detoxification system, a super family of enzymes called cytochrome P450. Exercise also increases the body's ability to remove activated carcinogens by increasing the activity of important binding compounds such as glutathione-S-transfer-ases that allow the body to safely excrete the toxins.

Because physical activity has such a profound effect on all five pathways, it could be even more important to cancer prevention than diet. Let's take a look at the intriguing scientific research in this area.

MYRIAD BENEFITS OF MOVEMENT

The American Cancer Society, the World Health Organization, the National Cancer Institute, and most respected leaders in the world of cancer prevention agree that physical activity can help prevent cancer. Why? Because scientific clinical studies have demonstrated that being physically active can reduce your risk of several cancers including breast, colon, uterine, and prostate. And there's even more good news—exercise has benefits that go way beyond cancer prevention.

BUILDS STRONG BONES. Many studies have shown that exercise can enhance the strength and density of our bones. A 2011 literature review from Florida State University confirms that aerobic exercise can serve as an effective nonpharmacological or complementary strategy to increasing and maintaining bone mineral density in older adults.

HERE'S TO YOUR HEART. The studies regarding the benefits of exercise to the cardiovascular system are numerous. It is now undisputed that regular physical activity can help enhance heart health by improving the condition of the heart, lowering blood pressure, and improving circulation. People engaged in regular exercise have a lower resting heart rate, decreased body mass index

(BMI), and lower blood pressure. These parameters of cardiovascular fitness are even more evident when the exercise is accompanied by weight loss.

HELPS PREVENT DIABETES. Exercise is believed to help prevent diabetes because it helps maintain a normal body weight. Numerous studies link physical activity with the prevention of diabetes and the maintenance of normal blood sugar levels. A 2010 literature review of five clinical randomized trials featured in the *Journal of Aging Research* focused on the benefits of resistance exercise on diabetes risk factors. All of the trials consistently demonstrated improvements in insulin signaling and reduction in both total and abdominal fat. The researchers concluded that resistance training "may play a role in improving the age-related increases in insulin-resistance and prevent the onset of diabetes."

MENOPAUSAL AT AGE 33! *By Karolyn*

Losing—and gaining—weight has been an issue for me for quite some time. Actually, it's the gaining that has been the "issue." I was operated on for ovarian cancer just two days after I turned 33. Following surgery, it was as if someone had flipped a switch and I was no longer Karolyn. So much had changed—my skin, my moods, and most notably my metabolism—virtually overnight. I have struggled with my weight ever since. I have been menopausal for more than 16 years!

But even though I struggle, I don't give up. I continually try new things. Most of all, I have learned that the only way I can stick with exercise is if I do the things I enjoy. I love to hike and horseback ride, so those are at the core of my program. I was intimidated by yoga, so I enlisted my friend Carrie to take a class with me. I have my setbacks, but I continue. Why? Not only because I know that it is helping to prevent a cancer recurrence, but mostly because it makes me feel better. Everything seems better when I am moving. My skin feels smoother, my mood improves, and I feel stronger—physically, emotionally, and even spiritually. Nearly all my physical activity is outside, and that certainly helps.

If you ever meet me in person, you will see that I am not rail thin. I am just me—someone who has finally figured out that exercise is more than just losing weight. It helps me thrive, and I love that!

MENTAL HEALTH MAGIC. Being physically active can improve your self-image, help you gain more confidence, reduce stress, and help you sleep better. That's mental health magic if you ask us! Many studies confirm the mental health benefits of exercise. Specific to cancer, a recent study from Georgetown University involving 192 people diagnosed with various cancers at various stages showed that higher rates of exercise were associated with lower rates of anxiety and depression and improved quality of life.

ENHANCES IMMUNITY. Several studies have shown that the strength of our immune system is directly influenced by physical activity. A 2009 study featured in *Exercise Sports Science Review* demonstrated that moderate-intensity exercise can help prevent respiratory tract viral infections and even reduce their duration.

POWERFUL CANCER PREVENTION. The research involving exercise and cancer prevention is most compelling for breast, prostate, and colon cancers. On the flip side, research shows a strong correlation with inactivity and increased risk of breast, colon, endometrial, kidney, esophageal, ovarian, rectal, and lung cancers. A comprehensive 2011 literature review featured in *Cancer Management and Research* looked at studies completed over the past decade and concluded that physical activity can help prevent several cancers and can benefit people previously diagnosed by helping to increase aerobic capacity, improve physical functioning, and contribute to overall quality of life. The researchers also stated that some of the most common side effects associated with cancer treatment can be alleviated through exercise. Many studies demonstrate exercise's benefit on recovery from cancer treatment and on restoring fitness after cancer treatment.

If you've had a previous diagnosis of cancer and are working hard to prevent a recurrence like we are, you will most definitely benefit from increased physical activity. A 2011 original report featured in the *Journal of Clinical Oncology* showed that men with a previous diagnosis of prostate cancer who were physically active had a significantly lower chance of dying of prostate cancer or any cancer. Those men who participated in vigorous activity (biking, tennis, jogging, swimming) for equal to or greater than three hours a week fared the best in terms of preventing a recurrence.

One of our favorite studies involving physical activity involves breast cancer. In this 2008 study, published in the *Journal of Clinical Oncology*, women who walked briskly at least two to three hours every week in the year before they were diagnosed with breast cancer were 31 percent less likely to die of the disease than women who were inactive before their diagnosis. This study also showed that women who **increased** their physical activity after their diagnosis had a 45 percent lower risk of death, while women who **decreased** their physical activity after their diagnosis had a four-fold greater risk of dying of cancer. Canadian researchers reported in *Recent Results in Cancer Research* that the benefits of physical activity specific to breast cancer are likely associated with a broad spectrum of effects that include controlling hormonal balance, insulin resistance, and chronic inflammation. We couldn't agree more. With the additional exercise-derived impacts on maintaining healthy body weight, improved digestion and detoxification, and enhanced mental health, you can begin to see why this is a powerful core component to our plan.

This is just the tip of the iceberg. The scientific data regarding the myriad benefits of exercise continue to be revealed. Knowing that exercise is good for you is the first step. The next step is to integrate regular physical activity into your daily life. In the next part of this chapter, we will provide practical information you can use to ramp up your physical activity and keep it ramped up.

FINDING THE RIGHT FIT

We've all heard that one person's trash is another person's treasure. Such is the case with physical activity as well. What one person enjoys, another may not. A person with serious animal allergies, for example, may not choose horseback riding as his primary form of physical activity. Someone who doesn't care for country music may not choose a line dancing class. But before we can even begin to explore what activities we may or may not like to do, we must first

"BUT I'M TOO BUSY TO EXERCISE"

Busting the Biggest Exercise Excuse Ever!

When we are busy, our fitness routine is often the first casualty of the day. This is ironic because exercise makes us more efficient and therefore less busy! Keeping a 30-minute "fitness appointment" can increase your overall daily work and home life efficiency dramatically. In addition, it will help you sleep better! The bottom line: The busier you get, the more you need to get physical. You can't afford not to exercise if you want to keep up the hectic pace of your life.

take an honest look at our individual fitness levels. What are we physically ready to do?

Please note that if you have been inactive for a while, you will want to get some direction from your health-care provider about starting a fitness program. Fitness trainers can also be helpful in creating a customized exercise program. Getting guidance early on in the process will ensure you are heading down the right path and will help you avoid frustration or, worse yet, an injury.

Let's start by loosely defining what it means to be physically active. The American Cancer Society (ACS) refers to this as "intentional activities," meaning fitness that is done above and beyond routine daily actions like walking to your car in the parking lot or going up and down stairs in your home. The ACS recommends that adults engage in at least 30 minutes of moderate to vigorous intentional activities at least five days a week. They note that 45 to 60 minutes is preferred.

Now that we have that straight, what is "moderate" and what is "vigorous"? Effort that is equal to a brisk walk is considered moderate. One way to know that you are walking briskly is if you are a bit breathless when you talk and have to catch your breath between sentences. Vigorous activities are generally defined as using large muscle groups such as in the legs, causing an increased heart rate, producing deeper and faster breathing, and encouraging sweating. If your friend says "I worked up a good sweat today," she was likely engaged in vigorous physical activity.

Look at it this way: A casual bike ride to the store is moderate unless you are riding fast because you need an ingredient for dinner—then it becomes a vigorous workout as you race against time. Ballroom dancing is a great moderate exercise, and doing the Samba can be fun vigorous exercise. Mowing the lawn is usually moderate exercise, whereas digging, carrying, and hauling to create a whole new yard is vigorous exercise. As your fitness level increases, it is important to transition from moderate to vigorous exercise as much as you can throughout the week. Keep in mind though that the initial objective is to just get moving.

GETTING STARTED

If you are presently not exercising regularly, the most important thing to keep in mind is to start slowly. Baby steps are the way to go. This may mean that you start by taking a five-minute walk every day. Once that becomes relatively easy, increase it to a 10-minute walk. Eventually, you can build up to three 10-minute walks daily. Over subsequent weeks, these short walks can be merged into one 30-minute walk daily. This is just one example of how to ease into a regular exercise program. Set goals and allow yourself time to get there.

This is especially true if you are significantly overweight. Exercising when you are carrying excess weight is not only more difficult, but it can be uncomfortable as well. In fact, obese individuals contemplating an exercise program often report they are afraid of getting injured, experiencing pain from exercise, and/or feeling embarrassed to exercise in public fitness centers. For all of these reasons, exercise can be particularly daunting for obese individuals.

It can also be difficult to start an exercise program if you are elderly, have arthritic joints, or have challenges with your eyesight or balance that make some forms of exercise difficult. Even if you fit into one of these categories, there are exercise programs that will work for you. Tai Chi, for instance, can be a very effective and fun way to regain strength, balance, and fitness. Tai chi is a system of gentle physical exercises and stretching movements. Tai Chi involves changing from one posture to another at a slow and deliberate pace. While the movement is constant, it is gentle and non-impactful to joints. One clinical study of older Chinese adults found that a 60-minute Tai Chi exercise class three times per week for 12 weeks improved balance, upper- and lower-body muscular strength, flexibility, and endurance in study participants. Tai Chi has also been shown to reduce fall risk in older adults and to improve overall quality of life.

If you are ready and able to engage in more vigorous exercise, one of the best ways to start is by walking. Investing in a good pair of walking shoes and comfortable work out clothing is important. As you become more conditioned, add in weight resistance training (more on this later). We agree with the ACS and other experts that a pedometer (a device that counts your steps) is a good investment, as it allows you to see how many steps you presently take and then work to increase that number. Most pedometers take a little bit of set up, but you can get help from personnel in running stores or fitness trainers. It takes about 2,000 steps to walk a mile. It's great if you can work up to 10,000 steps—or five miles—a day. Wearing a pedometer all day can be a fun way to stay active and to work toward a goal.

In addition to potentially investing in a pedometer, we also suggest you pay attention to where you are walking. We are big fans of doing as much exercise outdoors as possible. Studies show that exercising in nature—sometimes called "green exercise"— can have added benefits when compared to exercising indoors. A 2011 literature review featured in the journal *Environmental Science and Technology* asked the question: "Does participating in physical activity in outdoor natural environments have a greater effect on physical and mental wellbeing than physical activity indoors?" The answer? Yes, it does! After evaluating 11 studies including more than 800 adults, the researchers found that "exercising in natural environments was associated with greater feelings of revitalization and positive energy, decreases in tension, confusion, anger, and depression and increased energy." Further, they found

TOP FIVE FITNESS TIPS

1. **MOVE IN WAYS YOU ENJOY.** How do you move now, what do you imagine you would like to do, and what have you always wanted to try? It's important to make movement fun.

2. **WRITE DOWN YOUR FITNESS GOALS.** Why do you want to start moving in the first place? Are you at the point to take your activities to the next level? Having goals and checking in with those goals can help you stay motivated. Seek help from trainers and fitness experts if you are not sure what your goals should be.

3. **CREATE A ROUTINE.** Commit a time of day to exercise. Flexibility is important during exercise, but it isn't helpful when it comes to planning your exercise routine. Even if you have to adjust other things around your exercise time, it is worth it—you are worth it!

4. **START SOMETHING...ANYTHING.** If you haven't been physically active for a while you may feel like a stalled car. But remember, once you start pushing that car, it will build momentum, and you won't have to work as hard to keep it moving. And if you're lucky, your stalled car is at the top of a hill and your fitness routine will be off to a running start!

5. **KNOW YOUR STRENGTHS AND LIMITATIONS.** Do an honest assessment of your fitness level and choose activities that match that level. You may also need to consult with your doctor if you have not been physically active in a while. Set yourself up for success by creating a routine that is realistic and grows your fitness in small steps.

that people reported they were happier being physically active in nature and were more likely to repeat the activity. While we understand that it's not always possible to get outside while you exercise, we encourage you to do so whenever you can.

The key to regular exercise is to make sure that exercise is enjoyable. At first, the only thing that may get us moving is our understanding of the benefits of exercise. This sort of motivation, while handy on occasion, typically wears itself out after awhile. We need to be moti-

WHAT ABOUT YOGA?

Those who practice yoga will tell you that it is more than mere movement. In Sanskrit (the ancient language of India, where yoga originated), yoga means "union." To most people who do yoga, it is the uniting of mind, body, and spirit. Yoga provides the opportunity to focus on mental and spiritual well-being, as well as physical fitness. While yoga is the practice of physical postures and poses, the focus is on breath, movement, and being present.

Yoga is much more than stretching. It helps create balance in the body, enhancing flexibility as well as strength. There are several different types of yoga and you can participate no matter what level you are at. Even if you feel you are not flexible or strong, you can still benefit from yoga, because an individualized experience is created. Yoga is not about competing or achieving a certain result. Yoga is about developing your relationship with your body.

The health benefits associated with yoga have been studied extensively. Many of the studies involving cancer patients are small, but the results are compelling nonetheless. Recent research has focused on breast cancer survivors. In 2009, a randomized controlled trial involving 88 stage-II and -III breast cancer patients going through radiation therapy demonstrated that the women who participated in 60 minutes of yoga daily during the treatment had significantly fewer side effects such as anxiety, fatigue, insomnia, and appetite loss, compared to the women who did not do yoga.

A 2010 study showed that eight sessions of yoga combined with meditation and breathing exercises helped enhance perceived quality of life in women undergoing treatment for breast cancer. There was a statistically significant decrease in anxiety in the women who did the yoga.

In 2011, a pilot study involving breast cancer survivors showed that yoga significantly improved persistent fatigue, which is common among people who have gone through conventional cancer treatments. The women who completed the 12-week yoga program also reported better physical function, less depression, and enhanced overall quality of life.

A 2004 study featuring 39 patients with lymphoma demonstrated a significant improvement in sleep quality and duration. Participants who did yoga (with 58 percent completing at least five sessions) also reported decreased use of sleep medication and overall better sleep quality.

While many studies are looking at yoga to help people heal from cancer, there is good reason to believe that yoga can be a significant cancer prevention tool, as it enhances blood flow, improves mood, eases insomnia, and reduces stress.

vated to exercise because we enjoy it. There are many fun ways to move. Consider these options:

- Dancing to your favorite music
- Walking or running while listening to music or an electronic book
- Hiking on your favorite trail
- Bicycling on a bike path through picturesque areas
- Joining a recreational sports team
- Exercising with a friend
- Taking an exercise class or working with a trainer
- Trying something different like yoga or Tai Chi

There are many more options. The important thing is to experiment until you find activities that you enjoy and even look forward to. For many people, variety is also important. Doing different types of exercises will keep it interesting and help avoid boredom that can develop from having to repeat the same exercise over and over. Remember, exercise is movement, and movement should feel good on all levels—mental, emotional, and physical.

For more ideas, check out our Top Five Fitness Tips on page 79. By now you've figured out that you need to pick activities that you enjoy at least on some level, or you may not be able to sustain your exercise effort for long. You may also want to consult with a personal trainer or fitness expert to get an idea of your existing fitness level and get some input on appropriate fitness goals. In addition, to get optimum cancer protection, there are some other basics to keep in mind.

THE FITNESS FOUNDATION

While your fitness program should be unique to your individual likes and level, there are five core issues that every physical fitness program should include:

1. Muscle strengthening
2. Aerobic activity
3. Stretching and flexibility
4. Proper timing
5. Optimum hydration

Let's take a closer look at each of these.

MUSCLE STRENGTHENING. Did you know that every pound of muscle uses about six calories a day to sustain itself, whereas fat only burns about two calories a day? If you have more muscle, you will burn more calories and be better able to maintain a healthy weight. Muscle tone also helps prevent insulin resistance in the muscle itself, which is a primary source of insulin resistance systemically. Building muscle also increases our metabolism, which further helps us maintain healthy body weight and avoid insulin resistance.

When we think of strengthening or building muscle, we may first think about weight lifting. Lifting weights is an excellent way to condition muscles and is not reserved for bodybuilders alone. It is entirely appropriate for women to get just as comfortable in the free weight part of the gym as men. For people who would rather not work out with weights, there are many ways to condition muscles:

- Fast walking (you can wear ankle and wrist weights to build even more muscle)
- Jogging, running, or hiking
- Jumping rope
- Climbing stairs
- Doing push ups or jumping jacks
- Using resistance bands
- Practicing yoga

Weight-bearing exercises force the muscle to work against gravity or resistance. This action is what builds the muscle. Remember, when we work large muscle groups like the ones in the legs, we are participating in "vigorous" activity, which is the goal.

AEROBIC ACTIVITY. Large muscle groups are also significant with aerobic activity. To paraphrase the American College of Sports Medicine, aerobic exercise is an activity that uses large muscle groups, is done continuously, and is rhythmic in nature. The purpose is to cause the heart and lungs to work harder than when we are resting for an uninterrupted period of time. Some of the more well-known aerobic activities are running, bicycling, and swimming; however, dancing, jumping rope, cross country skiing, and in-line skating are also examples of aerobic exercise.

With consistent aerobic exercise, our bodies become conditioned, but if we don't vary the exercise, our muscles begin to lose some of that conditioning. If you've been doing the same type of aerobic activity, you could try to kick it up a notch. For example, if you are a brisk walker, try bursts of jogging for a few minutes during the course of your walk or hike. Inserting periods of more intense exercise within your normal workout is called interval training and enhances your aerobic conditioning. You can also try an entirely different type of exercise class or try the next level of aerobic classes.

STRETCHING AND FLEXIBILITY. It is important to keep your joints limber and your muscles stretched. This is a key component of any fitness program, and it also helps prevent injury. Gentle stretching after your muscles are warmed up and then after you are done exercising is ideal. Stretches should not be painful but should exert a continuous and noticeable pull on your muscles. Some types of physical activities such as yoga or Pilates incorporate stretching into the exercising itself. In fact, yoga and Pilates incorporate strength, aerobics, and flexibility as a part of the routine (for more information about yoga, refer to the side bar on page 80). Being more physically flexible can make everyday tasks easier. In addition to enhancing flexibility, stretching also improves balance, range of motion, and circulation. Stretching can also help relieve stress and prevent injury. Because stretching properly is critical, keep this in mind:

- Stretching should not be painful, so don't force yourself while stretching; you should only feel mild tension.

- Stretching should be fluid and gentle; don't bounce or throw your body into a stretch.

- Don't hold your breathe while stretching; use this as an opportunity to breathe freely and deeply.

- Stretch frequently throughout your day; in addition to stretching associated with exercise, you should also periodically stretch during the day and before you go to bed at night.

PROPER TIMING. Now for the fourth core issue, timing— after all, timing is everything right? Actually, it's not everything but it sure does mean a lot when it comes to physical activity. The first rule about fitness and timing is frequency. It is far better to do something more frequently (i.e., daily, even if for short durations) than to just exercise once or twice a week or on the weekends (the so-called weekend warrior). In order for your fitness program to be sustainable and to confer maximal health benefits, you need to build it into your daily routine. Make exercise a habit. Schedule it just as you would a daily conference call.

The other aspect of timing is when we exercise. Research has shown that people who exercise in the morning have a better chance of sustaining their activity in the long run. Moving in the morning can also help rev up your metabolism for hours afterward as you begin your day. This can lead to quicker benefits from the exercise, which may explain why people who exercise in the morning tend to stick with it. If you can't exercise in the morning, just be sure not to exercise too late at night. In general exercise helps with sleep, but if done too late in the evening it can have the opposite effect and keep you awake.

OPTIMUM HYDRATION. Dehydration may conjure images of a barren dessert and an isolated water mirage. However, dehydration begins long before we begin to feel parched. We'll discuss the many benefits of water in more detail in the cellular rejuvenation chapter, but it's important to emphasize the benefits of staying hydrated as our fifth core component of fitness. Even mild dehydration can slow down your body's metabolism and cause you to put on extra weight. On the other hand, increased consumption of water is associated with significant loss of body weight and fat. This has been demonstrated in several clinical studies of people who are overweight. One study randomly assigned 311 premenopausal, overweight (BMI 27–40) women aged 25 to 50 years, to a weight-loss diet. The researchers found that the women who increased their drinking water to at least one liter (just over four cups) each day had an additional five pounds of weight loss over 12 months. The weight loss was attributed to an increase in metabolism (energy expenditure at rest). Merely increasing water intake helps you burn fat! Drinking water also prevents you from confusing hunger with thirst, so you won't eat as much. Drink a glass of water before every meal or snack to help reduce the amount of calories you take in. This will also help you stay hydrated.

A small 2011 study from Missouri Western State University examined the effects of dehydration associated with resistance weight training in 10 healthy males. The researchers found that dehydration resulted in significantly lower repetitions, higher perceived exertion and heart rate, and hindered heart rate recovery. If you want to get the most of your fitness program—and the most out of your day for that matter—stay hydrated. Drink a minimum of eight, 8-ounce glasses of pure water every day.

Water that has been filtered by reverse osmosis and/or active carbon filtration is ideal. Avoid unfiltered tap water, as it has been shown to have harmful chemicals and even potentially cancer-causing agents. Water in plastic bottles with the numbers 2, 4, and 5 are the safest, as the plastic is less apt to leach cancer-causing bisphenols into the water. Plastic water bottles with number 1 imprinted on the plastic can be used one time only. Bottles with the numbers 3, 6, and 7 should be avoided. No matter how you drink your water, just be sure to drink sufficient amounts of it as part of your fitness program and your daily routine.

Whether you are choosing a round of golf, a hike, yard work, or a dance class, you should incorporate these five core practices into your routine: muscle strengthening, aerobic activity, stretching and flexibility, proper timing, and optimum hydration. For additional tips, refer to our top five fitness tips on page 79.

VARIETY IS THE SPICE OF LIFE

Remember in the last chapter when we discussed the importance of love, laughter, and joy? Well this is the perfect time to incorporate more of that into your weekly routine. Choose physical activities that you love. Exercise needs to be fun to be sustainable—or at least parts of it need to be fun. For example, some people may not have fun jogging, but they can make it more fun if they listen to music they enjoy or share the experience with a friend. Being physically active will not only help you prevent cancer, it will get you closer to being the healthy, vibrant person you were meant to be.

We were meant to move. To deny that is to deny who we really are on the deepest cellular level. The health benefits of having the courage and commitment to exercise will make the effort entirely worth it. And to embrace exercise does not mean we need to become an ironman or a marathoner. We need to get closer to what it means to us to be physical. Are you a gardener? Do you love the freedom of the open road on a bicycle? Do walks in the park with your four-legged best friend make you smile? Is it heading to the gym with a coworker, or maybe an early morning swim? You have lots of choices. Choose as many as possible, and get moving!

 **HIGH FIVE TIP** *The physical benefits of exercise are tremendous, but what you may not realize is that exercise is one of the most powerful antidepressants available. All types of exercise decrease depression. This is true for cancer survivors too. Researchers from Vanderbilt University and Shanghai Institute of Preventive Medicine found that women diagnosed with breast cancer who increased their exercise level after diagnosis had a 42 percent reduced risk for depression. You can strengthen the antidepressant effect of exercise by exercising more frequently and more vigorously. In general, more than two hours of exercise total per week will decrease depression.*

CHAPTER 5

HEALING FOODS

hether a person has had a previous cancer diagnosis or is trying to prevent cancer, we are often asked the same question: "What should I eat?" Implied in this question is the idea that there is one right answer. While there are some universally accepted principles, diets must be individualized in order to be most effective. Dietary individualization can, and should, occur over a lengthy time period so that a diet becomes a part of who we are and how we express ourselves in the world. If you were to adopt a dietary change overnight and declare that diet to be your new diet, it's highly unlikely you would sustain the changes for the long haul. Most of the time, our bodies and our psyches don't respond well to abrupt and dramatic change. Even when cancer is the motivator, dietary changes typically need to be put into place sequentially, and relentlessly, in order to be effective. Our Five to Thrive diet principles described in this chapter should be implemented with careful consideration and a high degree of patience. This will not only optimize your chance of success, it will give you time to get used to the diet and discover ways you can individualize it.

We believe diet is one of the most important components of our overall cancer prevention plan. Why is diet so important? Because it is the vehicle for obtaining the nutrients our bodies need to function. What we eat, how much we eat, and the way we eat dramatically influence the nutrition our cells receive. Therefore, the health and vitality of our bodies, on a cellular level, is directly determined by the state of our nutrition. As a result, diet is one of the most fundamental contributors to both health and disease.

WHAT'S THE PROOF THAT DIET AND LIFESTYLE WILL ACTUALLY PREVENT CANCER

Despite the immediate benefit of feeling healthier from changing your diet and lifestyle in the ways outlined in the Five to Thrive plan, you might still be holding out for proof that this plan will lower your risk of developing cancer. A study published in the April 2011 issue of *Cancer Epidemiology, Biomarkers & Prevention* makes the case pretty convincingly. The study analyzed diet and lifestyle questionnaires completed by 111,966 nonsmoking men and women in the Cancer Prevention Study II Nutrition Cohort. After 14 years, men and women with the highest compliance to diet and lifestyle habits aimed at maintaining a healthy body weight, eating a healthy diet that emphasized vegetable and fruit intake, limiting alcohol consumption, and exercising regularly had a 42 percent lower risk for death than those people who did not adhere to these healthy lifestyle habits. Risk for death from cardiovascular disease was 48 percent lower in men and 58 percent lower in women; risk for cancer death was 30 percent lower in men and 24 percent lower in women. The researchers concluded that a healthy diet and lifestyle that can be achieved in small steps over time does, in fact, lower the risk for cancer. The Five to Thrive plan provides practical, scientifically substantiated information with powerful tools to lower your risk of cancer—it's that simple.

MAKING THE CONNECTION

In terms of cancer, it is estimated that diet is responsible for 30 to 35 percent of all deaths from cancer. There are several ways we can understand the relationship between diet and cancer development. Probably the easiest way is to think of our diet as a source of fuel that our cells require to function. The higher the nutritional value of our diet, the more fuel we provide and the more optimally our cells will function. This is particularly relevant when you consider that at any given moment, millions of our cells are undergoing some form of either DNA damage or are battling the effects of epigenetic triggers that favor cancer development. To combat this cellular stress, we rely on the activity of our DNA repair and tumor suppressor genes. To perform their tasks effectively, these genes need nutrients. The job of these DNA repair and tumor suppressor genes is to provide the instructions to make proteins that do the actual cell repair and suppress abnormal cell activity and growth. Not only do we need the instructions to be correct, but we also need the proteins produced from these genes to be efficiently and accurately constructed. This construction process relies upon a steady flow of nutrients. Nowhere is the power of epigenetics more evident than it is here. The biochemical and nutrient soup in which our DNA and its proteins float determines the health and activity of these genes and their proteins. The molecular flavor of this biochemical soup is dependent upon the compounds obtained from our diet. Unfortunately, it's not always as straightforward as simply eating the nutrients required by either DNA or protein synthesis. This is because nutrients interact with one another and are metabolized and broken down into various active forms, and their activity inside cells changes depending upon other factors present. Given this high level of complexity, it's important to consider diet in terms of long-term, consistent impact.

Most cancers take years to develop. It makes sense, then, that the most effective cancer prevention diet is a diet that is sustained over years as well. This sustainability is a critical point. Consistently we hear people say they have difficulty sticking with some dietary changes. These highly motivated individuals, trying to do the right thing, embark upon ambitious dietary programs. But after a few months or even weeks, they become frustrated. As they struggle with their new diet, they often revert back toward a very unhealthy diet—almost as if to declare themselves incapable of eating well. "Why bother?" they ask us.

To be successful, a cancer prevention diet should have three key characteristics:

1. It must be scientifically substantiated and have scientific validation that it can, in fact, decrease the risk of cancer. It's not enough to have a theory; the diet must be validated through research.

2. It must be able to be maintained by the majority of people who try it—sustainability is critical. We have found that ex-

treme diets, while perhaps healthier or more beneficial for some individuals, are generally difficult to sustain. Because of this, these extreme diets do not constitute a realistic cancer prevention plan for most people. For example, many people would have difficulty converting to a raw foods diet and adhering to it long term. Likewise, taking all sugar, red meat, and dairy out of the diet, while healthy, may not be possible for some people—at least not overnight.

3. The diet must support the health of the key body pathways we've described: increased immunity, decreased inflammation, hormone balancing, decreased insulin resistance, optimal digestion and detoxification.

A diet that has these three characteristics is the ideal cancer prevention foundational diet.

CANCER LIKES EXCESS FAT

One of the goals of any cancer prevention diet should be to maintain an ideal body weight. Obesity is responsible for one in six cancer deaths in the United States. In the United States, obesity accounts for 14 percent of deaths from cancer in men and 20 percent of cancer-related deaths in women. Pay close attention: These percentages are directly related to dying of cancer. Excess weight increases the chance of dying of prostate cancer by 34 percent. Being overweight more than doubles the risk of dying of breast cancer. The current Western diet promotes excess weight with its predominance of refined sugar, simple carbohydrates, fat, and meat. These foods add weight, weaken immunity, and promote inflammation—all of which favor cancer growth.

Obesity has become a significant issue not just in the United States, but worldwide. According to the National Center for Health Statistics, in the period between 2005 and 2006, more than 67 percent of Americans between the ages of 20 and 74 were overweight. Between 1960 and 1962, that figure was just under 45 percent. This illustrates the alarming increase in obesity in a fairly short period of time. It's also an increase that is a very deadly trend. The impact

THE POWER OF FOOD *By Dr. Alschuler*

Julie (not her real name) was diagnosed with triple-negative breast cancer in her mid-40s. Triple negative breast cancer is unique because it does not express estrogen receptors, progesterone receptors or Her-2-neu receptors. Triple negative breast cancer can be aggressive and is considered more likely to recur and spread than other types of hormone dependent breast cancers. The lack of these receptors makes triple negative breast cancer more difficult to treat long term since hormonal therapies cannot be used. Despite the serious prognosis of this cancer, Julie underwent successful comprehensive and integrative treatment and is in her seventh year of being cancer-free.

Before her cancer diagnosis, Julie was not in the best of health. She had severe joint pain, depression, and significant digestive discomfort that caused her to experience daily bloating and constipation. Julie also had trouble sleeping. After she finished her chemotherapy, Julie decided she was ready to address her diet. After I assessed Julie's diet, I determined that she was likely sensitive to wheat gluten and ate significantly less vegetables and fruits than required. Over the next six months, Julie removed all wheat gluten from her diet. She did this by learning about wheat substitutes and experimenting with all types of foods that she could eat in place of her normal muffins, cookies, bread, and pasta. She eventually found foods that she enjoyed. At the same time, she increased her vegetable and fruit intake to six servings consistently every day.

Within the first six months of making these changes, Julie began to notice less joint pain, more energy, and better sleep. These improvements continued over the next year and she began to notice that she no longer felt depressed, her blood pressure was normalized, and she had fewer menopausal symptoms. As a result of these changes, Julie felt motivated to incorporate exercise into her lifestyle and began a program of daily walking. Even several years later, Julie is enjoying significantly better health and has remained cancer-free. She knew that she needed to make these changes gradually, one step at a time, in order for the changes to stick. The immediate benefits to her health, along with the knowledge that she is helping to prevent recurrence of her cancer, has made every plate of vegetables and every mile walked well worth it!

of obesity on cancer risk cannot be overstated. When choosing a diet, we must consider more than optimal nutrient intake. It is imperative that a cancer prevention diet include strategies to reverse obesity.

THE ART OF EATING

Before we go into more of the details about our cancer prevention diet, let's pause for a moment to discuss the simple act of eating. In our fast-paced, modern culture, we've lost touch with the greater significance of eating. If you think about it, eating is one of the most sensual experiences that we have. In fact, eating involves all of our senses. We entice our appetite by smelling food. The visual appearance of our food can make us ravenous or can evaporate our desire to eat. We touch food, both with our hands and with our mouths; the texture of food can stimulate digestion and be an enjoyable part of our eating experience. And, of course, we taste our food, which plays a fundamental role in determining the foods we prefer.

The sensuality of food is essential to our overall enjoyment of it, yet this is often the part of eating that our fast-paced culture causes us to neglect. How many times do we eat nondescript, tan-colored food out of a package that has no aroma and is bland in taste? The flip side is also true: People fill up on foods with artificial, inflated tastes—foods that are high in fat, sodium, and sugar—thus dulling the senses to the true flavor of "real" food. When we rely upon these meals, we are missing out on the wonderfully varied qualities naturally found in food. Unfortunately, these kinds of meals have become the norm for too many people. Over time, with the repetition of this monotonous experience of food, it is a natural reaction to lose the joy, wonder, and pleasure—the sensuality—of eating. When eating is no longer a sensual experience, we lose a critical component of our diet—that of complete *nourishment*.

Food supplies nutrients as well as nourishment. In fact, the act of eating is one of the most significant and direct ways we nourish ourselves. Caring enough about our health and our bodies to feed them properly is perhaps one of the most dramatic ways to rejoice in life and honor the human experience. Eating to nourish invokes health. Optimum health is built from appreciation for food and the ability to find pleasure in self-nourishment.

Our hope is that people who are motivated to use diet as a tool to help achieve greater health and prevent cancer will, in the process, experience a renewed sense of excitement. This excitement about eating is, fundamentally, an excitement about living. Feeding our bodies will only be satisfying when we are also feeding the spirit. Through diet, we can regain our sense of engagement with life and in so doing honor and feed the life force within us.

LASTING IMPACT

Imagine the difference between two hypothetical individuals, Jane and Joe. Jane has just recovered from treatment for early-stage breast cancer. Having gone through the difficulties of surgery and chemotherapy, she's motivated to make significant changes in her life to help prevent a cancer recurrence. She is so determined she joins a popular diet plan that provides optimal calories, increases vegetable intake, and minimizes excessive fats and sugars. On the surface this diet sounds good for Jane. True to the promises of the diet plan, four months later, Jane has lost eight pounds. During the fifth month, however, Jane's adherence to the diet begins to wane. She grows bored with the prepackaged meals, feels resentful she has to give up so much, and starts to fantasize about her favorite foods. Over the next several months Jane begins to slide off the wagon. If we fast-forward a couple years, we find that Jane has regained most of the weight—plus some additional pounds—and is no longer on the diet. She doesn't feel particularly motivated to try to lose weight or improve her diet because she now views all diets as difficult.

Now let's meet Joe. Joe has a family history of colon cancer and decides to make some changes to his diet. Joe realizes it's not a diet he's looking for; it's a lifestyle change that he can commit to and stick with. He decides to tackle one thing at a time. The first thing is to reduce his consumption of red meat, a previous staple of Joe's diet. He knows that heavy consumption of red meat is a significant risk factor for colon cancer. In the past Joe's wife did most of the cooking at home, but Joe has decided that for him to make this lifestyle change, he needs to play a more active role in the cooking. As he learns how to cook, Joe discovers the variety of spices and flavors available to him and the pleasure of preparing meals with color, aroma and flavor. He begins to develop a love of both wild-caught fish and organic chicken—great red meat alternatives. Eventually, Joe finds he no longer craves red meat. As Joe expands his culinary skills, he adopts additional healthful changes to his diet. In addition, he and his wife share the experience, which benefits their relationship.

OUR RECOMMENDATION REGARDING DETOXIFICATION DIETS

People often tell us—with pride—of the "brutal" detoxification or fasting type diet they undertake once or twice a year to totally cleanse their bodies. While these diets may have some benefit, they may also be jarring and inflammatory to the system. We believe in gentle detoxification throughout the year, which includes comprehensive support of our detoxification pathway. With its focus on whole foods, exercise, sleep, hydration, dietary supplements, and other aspects, the Five to Thrive diet and lifestyle plan does just that.

If you would like a more intense detoxification experience, periodically remove all processed foods, sugar, wheat and other refiend grains, and alcohol from the diet. Be sure you stay well hydrated to encourage daily bowel movements. Maintain this for three weeks for optimal benefit.

More comprehensive and sophisticated detoxification can be indicated for people with specific and known toxicities. Some people have high tissue levels of heavy metals or environmental chemicals that impair their health. These individuals will likely benefit from a tailored detoxification program developed by a naturopathic or integrative medical doctor with training in environmental medicine. It is important to undertake these types of detoxification programs under a doctor's guidance so the impacts on the body and the effectiveness of the detox can be assessed. Please note that aggressive detoxification following cancer treatment should only be undertaken under the supervision of a qualified healthcare provider. There are web sites listed in the resource section that will help you find a healthcare professional in your area.

Remember, ongoing detoxification can take place every moment of every day with the support of the Five to Thrive plan.

When asked about his diet, he describes it with enthusiasm, joy, and great satisfaction. And even more important, Joe feels better and is confident he is well on the way to preventing cancer.

These scenarios illustrate the importance of sustainable dietary change. The key is to improve nutritional quality while enhancing enjoyment. Remember, it's not about adhering to a "diet," it's about establishing a way of life. Yes, we may make choices that are not always the best, but we have countless opportunities to make different choices next time. For example, there may be an occasion when we order a piece of chocolate cake instead of a berry sorbet. In the morning, you may grab a cheese Danish instead of having a bowl of oatmeal. The worst thing we can do when we make a choice that is perhaps not the healthiest is to beat ourselves up and feel guilty about it. When we reprimand ourselves too harshly, we not only suffer the negative nutritional consequences of our choice, we also experience the added emotional burden. There is an enormous body of research linking emotions such as guilt, depression, and anger with weakened immune function, increased inflammation, and general poor health.

The good news is that every time we make a choice about what we eat, we create an opportunity to start fresh. Regardless of the choices we've made previously, every meal or snack gives us the chance to build and renew our health. This is not to say we should ignore our diet or repeatedly eat things we know will contribute to poor health. We have found that the more frequently we make sound dietary choices, the more quickly it will become second nature. As a part of the process, it's important to understand why we make the choices we make. For some people, choosing that Danish instead of oatmeal may simply be the result of not having sufficient time in the morning to make oatmeal. In this instance, the healthy response is to examine the morning ritual in order to create more time to prepare the oatmeal or replace the oatmeal with something quick and healthy, like fruit and yogurt. There are a number of reasons we make the choices we make. It's important to pause long enough to understand those reasons. With this understanding comes the opportunity to make healthier choices next time.

THE FIVE TO THRIVE DIET PLAN

In keeping with these concepts of gradual, deeply fulfilling dietary changes, the Five to Thrive diet plan is purposefully simple and straightforward, and yet holds the promise of a renewed sense of enjoyment from food. As you may have expected, there are five key premises of our diet plan:

1. Consume sufficient calories, but not excessive calories.

2. Eat a colorful diet.

3. Eat a whole-foods diet.

4. Emphasize plant and marine sources of fat.

5. Reduce or eliminate refined, processed, and packaged foods.

Let's take a closer look at all five components, beginning with quantity versus quality. **The first Five to Thrive diet premise is eating enough but not too much.**

Ancient Roman author Cicero was quoted as saying "...let moderation be your guide." The American diet has become the antithesis of Cicero's advice—it is the perfect example of lack of moderation. Eating sufficient calories but not eating in excess has become increasingly difficult in our modern world as the portion size most Americans consider normal far exceeds what we actually need to maintain health. Protein is a good example. An optimal serving of protein for most people is three to four ounces, or the size of a deck of cards. Imagine how you would feel if you went out to eat, ordered a meat dish from the menu, and were served a portion the size of a deck of cards. Most people would be shocked and would complain to the manager, even though that portion is just the right size based on what our bodies need. How about complex carbohydrates? A healthy serving of complex carbohydrates, or whole grains would be one slice of whole wheat, rye, or other whole-grain bread; one-half cup of whole-grain cereal; or one-half cup of cooked, whole-grain pasta. Think of the last time that you sat down to a bowl of pasta. Was it more than a half-cup? Chances are it was. While it is important to eat whole grains, and a healthy diet includes three to six servings of whole grains every day, many people consume that in one meal. We simply overeat.

BODY MASS INDEX (BMI) CHART

BMI (kg/m²)	19	20	21	22	23	24	25	26	27	28	29	30	35	40
Height (in.)	Weight (lb.)													
58	91	96	100	105	110	115	119	124	129	134	138	143	167	191
59	94	99	104	109	114	119	124	128	133	138	143	148	173	198
60	97	102	107	112	118	123	128	133	138	143	148	153	179	204
61	100	106	111	116	122	127	132	137	143	148	153	158	185	211
62	104	109	115	120	126	131	136	142	147	153	158	164	191	218
63	107	113	118	124	130	135	141	146	152	158	163	169	197	225
64	110	116	122	128	134	140	145	151	157	163	169	174	204	232
65	114	120	126	132	138	144	150	156	162	168	174	180	210	240
66	118	124	130	136	142	148	155	161	167	173	179	186	216	247
67	121	127	134	140	146	153	159	166	172	178	185	191	223	255
68	125	131	138	144	151	158	164	171	177	184	190	197	230	262
69	128	135	142	149	155	162	169	176	182	189	196	203	236	270
70	132	139	146	153	160	167	174	181	188	195	202	207	243	278
71	136	143	150	157	165	172	179	186	193	200	208	215	250	286
72	140	147	154	162	169	177	184	191	199	206	213	221	258	294
73	144	151	159	166	174	182	189	197	204	212	219	227	265	302
74	148	155	163	171	179	186	194	202	210	218	225	233	272	311
75	152	160	168	176	184	192	200	208	216	224	232	240	279	319
76	156	164	172	180	189	197	205	213	221	230	238	246	287	328

TIPS FOR REDUCING PORTION SIZE

- Use smaller plates and bowls.
- Serve yourself 75 percent of what you think you want.
- When eating out, ask for smaller portions.
- Eat slowly, putting your eating utensil down between each bite. This will allow your stomach to fill up with less food.
- If dining out with a companion, suggest splitting an entree.
- Drink a large glass of water before going back for more.
- Eat smaller meals more often in order to avoid becoming excessively hungry and binging.

One of the answers to this overconsumption challenge is to institute portion control. Portion control is critical to a healthy cancer prevention diet. As with any dietary change, it's best to implement this over time. If you were to reduce your portion sizes by half tomorrow, you probably wouldn't be able to stick with it. In the days and weeks that follow, your portions would likely creep back up to where they started. Part of this is physiological. The stomach increases its stretching capacity depending upon the size of meals we eat. If we are in the habit of consuming large quantities of food, the stomach accommodates those meals. Over time, the stomach enlarges, and hunger signals are generated if the stomach is not adequately filled. Because we tend to eat when we are hungry, reducing our portions too quickly would not allow time for the stomach to shrink. It is much more effective to gradually cut portion size and allow the body's physiology to change over time rather than expect it to change overnight. If we reduce portion size over the course of weeks, our stomachs will shrink and eventually we will feel satisfied with less food.

HOW MUCH FOOD DO WE NEED?

What is the optimal quantity of food? It depends on the person. A physically active 185-pound male requires more food each day to maintain his ideal health than a 115-pound, sedentary female. Age, exercise frequency, overall health, and genetics influence how much food we need. That means that any generalizations may only be partially accurate. The following guidelines are just that—guidelines—and will help you determine what is ideal for you.

The Harris Benedict equation, originally developed in 1919, is used to determine caloric requirements based on your sex, basal metabolic rate (BMR), and activity level (http://www.bmi-calculator.net/bmr-calculator/harris-benedict-equation/The Harris). This equation is useful in determining optimal caloric intake for people who are close to their ideal weight. However, for obese individuals or highly muscular individuals (e.g., body builders), this formula is not as accurate. For these individuals, a consultation with a qualified healthcare practitioner, such as a dietician or nutritionist, will help to determine ideal caloric intake. An adult who has a body mass index (BMI) of 30 or higher is considered obese. To calculate your BMI, go to www.bmi-calculator.net or refer to the chart on page 97.

It is much easier to count calories nowadays with the advent of various food and fitness applications for smart phones and computers. Many of these "apps" are often free and will provide the full nutritional profile of foods that you input or that you scan in by the bar code on the packaging. These programs will also keep track of your daily caloric intake as you progress towards your goal. Tools like this can make a dedicated weight loss effort much easier.

As a rule, sustained weight loss is best accomplished by cutting about 500 calories from your daily diet every month until you achieve your optimal caloric intake level. In addition to reducing calorie consumption, you should also focus on expending more calories through physical activity. The combination is most effective for losing weight. It is important to always obtain a sufficient minimum amount of calories. In general, women should not consume less than 1,200 calories each day, and men should not consume less than 1,800 calories per day.

QUALITY OVER QUANTITY

Now that we have figured out how much to eat, let's learn about what to eat. **The second premise of the Five to Thrive diet is to consume colorful foods.** Why is this so important? Because more than 200 large population studies have shown that people who eat colorful fruits and vegetables are less likely to get cancer. Regular consumption of different colors and types of fruits and vegetables ensures a consistent supply of a variety of nutrients that have potent anticancer actions. These powerful nutrients are called phytonutrients (*phyto* meaning plant).

More than 25,000 different phytonutrients in plant-based foods have been identified as having anticancer effects. These phytonutrients help support the five pathways on a cellular level to help prevent cancer. These nutrients represent a wide array of diverse compounds, including flavonoids and polyphenols. These compounds are pigmented and are responsible for the diverse natural colors in fruits and vegetables. That is why eating a colorful diet ensures a synergistic array of cancer-fighting nutrients.

You will want to remember the term *flavonoids*. This group of phytonutrients has emerged as being absolutely critical to cancer prevention. Flavonoids have potent antioxidant activity. Antioxidants neutralize reactive, or oxidative, compounds that are produced as a result of tissue damage from sunlight, radiation, infection, and chemicals, as well as from metabolic processes such as breathing, eating, and moving. If our cells lack sufficient antioxidants, then these reactive compounds cause extensive cell and organ damage and ultimately disease. Our cells produce some of our antioxidants and we obtain other antioxidant benefits from foods—particularly fruits and vegetables. More than 4,000 naturally occurring flavonoids have been identified in fruits and vegetables. Many animal and preclinical studies using human cells have shown that these compounds protect cells against oxidative damage that can otherwise lead to diseases including cancer. Studies also demonstrate that there is power in having a variety of these compounds rather than high quantities of a single compound. This is the rationale for consuming a diet with an array of vegetables and fruits, because this variety will ensure a constant supply of thousands of different phytonutrients, even if they are present in small quantities. A lifetime of consuming a variety of fruits and vegetables will help protect cells against becoming cancerous. In fact, people with a low intake of fruits and vegetables have a twofold-increased risk of developing cancer. The protective effect of flavonoids against cancer has been demonstrated for all cancer types. What's more, variety really is the spice of life when it comes to fruits and vegetables because there is a beneficial synergistic effect. Studies have shown that when several fruits are eaten together, the combined antioxidant activity is much greater than when the same quantity of a single fruit is eaten. Most studies demonstrate protection against cancer when people consume five to 10 servings of fruits and vegetables every day.

Another benefit of a colorful diet is that the variety stimulates your different taste receptors. In other words, a flavorful, colorful diet is more likely to taste good, which bodes well for that sustainability factor that we previously emphasized. While a discussion about all of the different phytochemicals found in fruits and vegetables and the various ways that they exert cancer-prevention actions would require far too many pages, we can offer a brief illustration of how a few of these powerful compounds can help prevent cancer.

Perhaps you've heard the term *polyphenols* in association with grape juice or red wine. Polyphenols, namely anthocyanins, are colorful compounds found in the skins of most berries including blueberries, strawberries, cherries, raspberries, blackberries, and grapes. Anthocyanins are important compounds because they exert potent antioxidant activities by binding to reactive oxidative molecules, thereby preventing these molecules from damaging our cells. Anthocyanins are also important because they have powerful anti-inflammatory actions. One of the key modulators of inflammation inside our cells is a gene called nuclear factor kappa B, (NF-kB). NF-kB can be thought of as the master switch of inflammation inside our cells. As we mentioned, people with chronic inflammation are at increased risk for the development of cancer. One of the characteristics of chronic inflammation is elevated NF-kB activity. In one study, anthocyanins in the form of bilberry extract (300 mg) consumed daily for three weeks reduced the activation of NF-kB by up to 45 percent in humans. A study published in *Clinical Experimental Metastasis* journal found that polyphenols in grapes inhibit NF-kB activity and proliferation of metastatic breast cancer cells when given orally to mice at doses equivalent to typical daily doses in humans. These are just a couple of the many studies that demonstrate the potent anti-inflammatory effects of polyphenols.

SPICE UP YOUR LIFE!

One of the ways you can enhance the eating experience is by tapping into your senses, and there is nothing more satisfying than the aroma and taste of colorful spices. As we mentioned, spices are a great source of polyphenols—health-promoting, cancer-fighting compounds. But more than that, spices are flavorful, aromatic and appealing to the eye. Some of our favorite tasty anticancer spices include turmeric (curcumin), oregano, rosemary and garlic.

When it comes to garlic, some people are deterred by the odor. Garlic supplements are a good alternative if dietary garlic isn't appealing. We recommend aged garlic extract that comes from 100% organic garlic bulbs (Kyolic®). There is also more information about these polyphenol rich supplements in Chapter 7, including a special form of curcumin from turmeric (BCM-95®). It can be difficult to achieve a therapeutic dosage of curcumin through diet alone, so supplementation is highly recommended. In health food stores look for CuraMed or ask your doctor about CuraPro. Both of these products contain BCM-95.

Remember, dietary supplements are meant to supplement your diet, not take the place of healthful foods. Be sure to spice up your life—and enhance your health in the process—by adding more spices to your daily meals.

In addition to their anti-inflammatory actions, polyphenols also reduce insulin resistance. A study featured in the *Journal of Nutrition* demonstrated that having a smoothie containing 2/3 cup of blueberries twice a day for six weeks significantly improved insulin sensitivity in obese individuals. This is no surprise: Berries have been shown to increase insulin sensitivity and lower blood sugar. This is likely due to the fact that berries are one of the richest sources of polyphenols—right up there with certain spices and dried herbs, cocoa products, flaxseeds, nuts (chestnut, hazelnut), some vegetables like globe artichoke heads, olives, and olive oil. Be sure to buy organic berries whenever you can in order to avoid exposure to pesticide residues.

Polyphenols reduce inflammation, provide antioxidant effects, protect DNA against damage, improve the health of insulin receptors thereby reducing insulin resistance, and positively influence many of the key hormonal pathways in the body. These healthy actions are the result of hundreds of polyphenol flavonoids, including:

- Curcumin from turmeric

- Carnosol from rosemary

- Epigallocatechin gallate (EGCG) from green tea

- Resveratrol from grapes

- Quercetin from citrus fruits and onions

- Sulforaphane from broccoli

This list is just the tip of the iceberg. Remember there are thousands of polyphenols found in fruits and vegetables. And the good news is that research shows us that each polyphenol has multiple health-promoting effects within the body. With thousands of polyphenols in the world, it makes sense that there are thousands of studies demonstrating the many anti-cancer actions of these phytonutrients. Focusing on dietary polyphenols is important. While supplementation of individual polyphenols such as curcumin, sulforaphane, or resveratrol may be helpful, it is critical that the foundation of prevention lie within the diet.

This brings us back to color. When we consume a variety of colorful fruits and vegetables, we are assured of consuming the different polyphenols, flavonoids, and other nutritional compounds that are critical to cancer prevention. These compounds modulate the activity of more than 500 and likely thousands of genes, which in turn creates multiple and complex effects that cumulatively promote healthy cell growth and behavior, thus helping to prevent cancer development. If you only remember one thing about our cancer prevention diet, remember this: the more color, the better!

The third premise of the Five to Thrive diet plan is to eat whole, and preferably organic, foods. By whole foods we mean foods that appear on your plate much like they looked when they were plucked from the earth. Whole foods are minimally processed, so the nutrients they contain are largely intact when you eat them.

Organic fruits and vegetables frequently have the highest nutrient content, containing more of those beneficial polyphenols, vitamins, and minerals than the conventionally grown alternative. At the 2009 Ecofarm Conference, Charles Benbrook, PhD, chief scientist with The Organic Center (www.organic-center.org), presented an evaluation of 236 studies that collectively demonstrated that organic foods were nutritionally superior to conventionally grown foods 61 percent of the time. According to a paper published in 2010 by Walter J. Crinnion, ND, in *Alternative Medicine Review*, multiple studies confirm the information that Benbrook presented. Crinnion reported that in addition to having fewer toxic chemicals, organic foods had greater nutritional value—especially significantly greater levels of vitamin C, iron, magnesium, phosphorus, and antioxidant phytonutrients. Organic foods also support our health by creating a healthier environment. Organically grown vegetables and fruits are not exposed to cancer-causing pesticides, herbicides, and synthetic fertilizers. This third Thrive recommendation is about getting back to basics. By focusing on whole, unprocessed foods, we are more fully nourishing our bodies and putting less strain on our detoxification pathway.

Whole grains are a great example of a "whole" food. Grains such as whole wheat, brown rice, barley, millet, quinoa, and oats can all be eaten as unprocessed, unrefined grains. In their unprocessed, whole form, these grains are rich sources of antioxidant compounds, fiber, vitamins, and minerals. Whole grain intake is associated with reduced risk of several cancers, including digestive tract, breast, ovarian, prostate, bladder, kidney, lymphoma, leukemia, and others. In large population studies, intake of whole grains has been shown to reduce the risk of cancer by as much as 70 percent. One of the reasons whole grains have such important cancer-prevention effects is due to their anti-inflammatory properties. In a study published in the journal *Breast Cancer Research and Treatment*, fiber intake was found to reduce C-reactive protein (CRP), a marker of inflammation in breast cancer survivors. Women who consumed 15.5 grams per day of dietary insoluble fiber were 49 percent less likely to have elevated CRP. The researchers concluded that a diet high in fiber (close to 20 grams per day) is associated with lower concentrations of CRP and therefore decreased inflammation. A reduction in systemic inflammation increases the likelihood of long-term cancer-free survival.

In addition to whole grains, a whole foods diet also contains other unprocessed or minimally processed foods, such as meat from organically fed, free-ranging animals; organic eggs; and of course fruits and vegetables. We understand that some individuals choose not to eat any form of animal-based protein for personal, philosophical, or health reasons. However, for others these foods can be helpful inclusions in a cancer prevention diet as long as they are sourced from organically, preferably grass-fed, free-ranging animals (for more information on dairy, refer to the Q&A section beginning on page 112).

Animal foods tend to be dense sources of protein, and protein is essential for immune function, optimal detoxification, and hormonal balance. It is true, however, that protein from commercially fed animals is relatively unhealthy food. Commercially fed beef tends to contain high quantities of saturated fat and can have residual antibiotics, pesticides and other cancer-causing compounds. Conversely, free-range, grass-fed beef tends to have a fatty acid ratio similar to that of fish—including increased polyunsaturated fats. Grass is a rich source of polyunsaturated fatty acids, so tissues in cows eating grass will be composed of more polyunsaturated fats. When we eat meats from grass-eating animals, we then obtain meat with a greater concentration of polyunsaturated fats. These fats are anti-inflammatory, immune supportive, and are associated with decreased cancer risk.

A randomized, double-blinded, dietary intervention study compared 20 healthy subjects who consumed three portions per week of red meat (beef and lamb) from either grass-fed animals or commercially fed animals. After four weeks, blood samples taken from these subjects revealed that the concentration of omega-3 polyunsaturated fatty acids was significantly higher in those subjects who consumed red meat from grass-fed animals. Grass-fed beef, particularly when prepared with a marinade of antioxidant spices such as ginger, rosemary, tumeric, or garlic, can be a healthy way to obtain sufficient protein and calories. A spice marinade reduces the formation of the heterocyclic amines that are formed when animal meat is exposed to high heat. Heterocyclic amines are cancer-causing compounds. By marinating meat with antioxidant spices such as those mentioned previously, cooking meat rare to medium rare, and avoiding charring the meat, you reduce heterocyclic amine formation.

The fatty acid profile of animal protein is a critical factor. Excess consumption of saturated and trans fats, which are found in commercially fed beef, high-fat dairy products, and other processed and packaged foods, are associated with increased risk of various cancers including breast, prostate, pancreatic, and colon. Consumption of a diet high in saturated fat results in a proinflammatory "obesity-linked" gene expression profile. Conversely, a diet that contains more polyunsaturated and monosaturated fats creates an anti-inflammatory gene profile. This was demonstrated in a clinical trial of 20 people with metabolic syndrome (a combination of insulin resistance and cardiovascular disease). This trial found that the consumption of virgin olive oil, a health-promoting source of monosaturated fat, turned off several pro-inflammatory genes and, in so doing, reduced markers of inflammation and metabolic syndrome. When virgin olive oil is the main source of dietary fat, the long-term anti-inflammatory effects can be significant and can lower the risk for inflammatory diseases, including cancer. Monosaturated fat is found in high percentage in olive oil, avocados, and macadamia nuts. This is epigenetics in action—dietary factors influencing the behavior of our genes and altering our state of health.

This brings us to the fourth premise of the Five to Thrive diet plan: increased consumption of foods containing essential fatty acids (EFAs). Polyunsaturated fats are essential fatty acids found in all vegetables, fish, seeds, and nuts. The majority of polyunsaturated fats occur as omega-6 fatty acid, also known as linoleic acid (LA). A plant-based diet will typically have sufficient omega-6 fatty acids. However, omega-3 fatty acids, including alpha-linolenic acid (ALA), eicosapentaenoic acid (EPA), and docosahexaenoic acid (DHA), are not as easy to get from diet unless you know where to find them. Good sources of ALA are flaxseeds, chia seeds, and hemp seeds. EPA and DHA are found in algae and fish (notably deep-sea fish such as cod, halibut, and salmon, but also in smaller fish like anchovies, herring, mackerel, and sardines). Fats should constitute no more than 30 percent of your diet, but even more important than percentage is the type of fat that's in the diet. Some fats are good for you, like essential fatty acids; however, some fats are bad for your health and can actually damage the five key pathways. When we eat the wrong types of fat or too much fat, we compromise our immunity, increase inflammation, disrupt hormonal communications, and increase obesity—all key risk factors for developing cancer.

This is important for vegetarians too, as the choice of vegetables and vegetable oils has significant impact on the overall fatty acid profile in our cells. As an example, dietary canola oil decreases colon cancer risk, whereas dietary corn oil increases the risk. This is because corn oil has higher levels of omega-6 fatty acids, whereas canola oil has higher omega-3 fatty acids. In animals fed canola oil, inflammatory markers such as COX-2 are significantly lower than in animals fed corn oil. Another concern for vegetarians is that EPA and DHA are only found in fish and algae, so algae-sourced EPA and DHA supplements may be necessary.

It is important to consume a sufficient amount of omega-3 fatty acids, specifically EPA and DHA. Consumption of these two EFAs has been shown to increase apoptosis (cell death) and decrease proliferation of pre-cancerous cells. These fats are called "essential," because the body cannot produce them—so it's essential to get them through the diet. Omega-3 essential fatty acids are incorporated into cell membranes, making the cells more fluid and less susceptible to oxidative damage, insulin resistance and inflammation. A diet concentrated in omega-3 fatty acids increases insulin sensitivity and controls blood glucose levels. Omega-3 fatty acids also improve immune function, specifically by increasing the ability of the immune system to recognize and destroy mutated cells. An omega-3–rich diet promotes anti-inflammatory cellular pathways, ultimately increasing the body's resistance to the inflammatory effects of various stressors. People who obtain a high percentage of their fats from EPA and DHA have lower risk of breast, prostate, and colon cancers because these fats positively influence all five pathways.

While increasing consumption of healthy fats, it is important to decrease consumption of unhealthy fats. There are two types of unhealthy dietary fats: trans fats and saturated fats. Trans fats are the most dangerous fat of all. They are created synthetically via high heat in a process known as hydrogenation. Foods containing trans fats should be avoided completely, even though it can be difficult. The U.S. Food and Drug Administration allows foods with less than 0.5 grams of trans fats per serving to be labeled as containing zero grams of trans fat. This means that a food with as much as 0.49 grams of trans fat per serving will not have trans fat appear on the label. By manipulating the serving size, foods can appear to be trans fat–free, when in reality the commonly eaten quantity has signifi-cant amounts of trans fats. So while it is important to read labels carefully, the most fail-proof way to avoid synthetic trans fats is to avoid processed foods. Trans fats are found in breakfast cereals, packaged pastries, cookies, bars, crackers and most fast foods.

Saturated fats are found in animal products. As mentioned pre-viously, we can minimize our ingestion of saturated fats if we eat animal products that come from grass-fed, free-ranging animals. The healthiest diet eliminates trans fats, reduces saturated fats, and increases essential fatty acids. And the most important group of EFAs is omega-3 fatty acids. You can see why this piece of dietary advice becomes an "essential" part of the Five to Thrive diet plan.

Number five of the Five to Thrive diet plan is to reduce con-sumption of refined, processed, and packaged foods. Refined foods are those that have been milled or processed in such a way as to remove their nutritional content. Some examples of refined foods include white flour, table sugar, and white rice. Refined foods are typically the main component of convenience foods and have become a prominent part of the Western diet. For this reason, it can be difficult to remove refined foods entirely from one's diet. How-ever, it's absolutely critical that we reduce refined foods as much as possible. Here's why.

Processed foods include foods that have been chemically altered in such a way as to increase the ability to mass-produce and preserve these foods. These foods have low nutritional content and contain synthetic or chemical additives that put a strain on the detoxification pathway. How do you know if a food is highly processed? Look at the label, and if the ingredient list contains long, difficult to pronounce words, then it's quite likely that the food is highly processed. The more "unnatural" the ingredients, the more likely the food will be harmful to your health. Many of the chemical additives, food dyes, and preservatives found in packaged and processed foods are inflammatory compounds and are therefore associated with increased risk of cancer.

Not only are refined and processed foods devoid of nutrients—meaning the calories they provide are "empty"—but they also promote inflammation, suppress immune function, increase insulin resistance, increase the production of stress (pro-inflammatory) hormones, and can impair digestion and detoxification. As you can see, there's no real health benefit to refined foods. In fact, just the opposite is true, as these foods impair the health of each of the five key pathways that are so critical to cancer prevention. Even one meal of refined carbohydrates significantly increases NF-kB activity, encouraging the inflammatory response. Refined grains lack fiber to slow their absorption and as a result, eating refined carbohydrates causes spikes in blood sugar. Over time, these blood-sugar spikes strain the pancreas and ultimately can contribute to insulin resistance. An occasional snack of refined grains is unlikely to cause long-term health issues; however daily consumption of refined and processed foods unravels our health. Take time this week to evaluate the amount of processed foods you eat. Fortunately, there are many natural alternatives now available to replace these processed foods in order to keep their consumption to an absolute minimum.

You will also find highly processed and unhealthy foods at fast-food restaurants. In addition to highly processed foods, these restaurants feature a lot of fried food options. High heat frying (such as with French fries, chicken wings, etc.) creates substances called acrylamides, which are known to cause cancer. In our presentations we have a slide that reads, "If you have to drive through to get it, keep driving!" We realize it may be difficult to avoid fast food entirely with today's hectic lifestyle; however, it's absolutely critical to reduce your consumption considerably. Start out slowly. For example, if you eat fast food three times a week, make a commitment to only go once a week, then every other week, and then only once a month. Trust us, you won't miss the drive through line.

A FEW DAYS IN THE LIFE OF THE FIVE TO THRIVE DIET

	Meals	Food	Total Daily Serving
Day 1	Breakfast	Oatmeal with blueberries, raw almonds, and agave nectar	3 servings fruit
	Lunch	A large bowl of mixed vegetable salad with a grilled chicken breast and olive oil–based salad dressing	5 servings vegetables 2 serving nuts 3–5 servings whole grains
	Dinner	Tofu, mushroom, onion, cashew, ginger, garlic stir-fry in olive oil with brown rice	3 servings protein
	Snacks	Apple, trail mix, 2 oz chocolate	
Day 2	Breakfast	Fresh fruit, flaxseed meal, and protein powder shake	3 servings fruit
	Lunch	Egg salad, lettuce, and tomato sandwich on whole-wheat bread with vegetable soup	6 servings vegetables 1 serving seed
	Dinner	Chicken and mixed vegetable coconut milk curry over quinoa	4 servings whole grains
	Snacks	Tortilla chips and guacamole	4 servings protein
Day 3	Breakfast	2 hard boiled eggs, whole-grain toast, and an orange	2 servings fruit
	Lunch	Black beans and rice with a side of steamed kale	5 servings vegetables 2 servings legumes
	Dinner	Halibut, asparagus, and sweet potato	4 servings whole grains
	Snacks	Strawberries with dark chocolate sauce	3 servings protein

Also, be mindful of what you order at those restaurants. If you normally get a large soda pop, cut it back to a small. Order the salad instead of fries, or get the grilled chicken instead of the fried fish. Or try a sub shop instead of a cheeseburger joint. Every little change you make will get you closer to your ultimate goal of avoiding processed, unhealthy foods entirely.

If you have a specific dietary question that has not yet been answered, refer to the "Common Diet Questions" below.

LET'S REVIEW

Our plan is a foundational cancer prevention diet—it is a shift in lifestyle, a different way of thinking and feeling about food. At the core of the Five to Thrive plan is the importance of enjoyment. Part of that enjoyment comes from broadening our food intake to include a variety of whole, naturally colorful foods and flavorful spices. Eating sufficient quantities, but limiting excess consumption, is a core component. Concentrate on a plant-based diet with a minimum of five to 10 servings of fruits and vegetables every day. Avoid refined, processed, and packaged foods in order to avoid empty calories and potentially harmful substances. Focus on essential fats from vegetables and fish. And, best of all, there are only five things to focus on so you don't have to worry about adhering to extreme changes or radical diets that can become overwhelming.

COMMON DIET QUESTIONS

Following is a compilation of some of the most common diet questions we've been asked over the years. Chances are, there may be one or two of these questions that you've been wondering about.

Q: Can I or should I eat soy?

A: Soy foods and the isoflavones they contain have been shown in many studies to be potent anticancer compounds. In populations in which soy intake is a main part of the diet, such as in many Asian countries, the incidence of most cancers is lower than in populations that don't consume soy. Furthermore, when people from those Asian countries move to Western countries and adopt a Western diet that has little to no soy, their rates of cancer increase to the same rates of their Western counterparts. Additionally, epidemiological studies have shown that soy consumption can reduce the risk of developing various cancers, including cancers of the prostate and breast.

Despite this data, many women have been instructed to avoid soy if they have a history of estrogen receptor positive (ER+) breast cancer. This is because soy contains compounds known as phytoestrogens that can bind to estrogen receptors and therefore theoretically could stimulate those estrogen receptors much in the same way that estrogen does, thereby accelerating the growth of estrogen-dependent cancers. However, several clinical trials of women with a history of breast cancer have demonstrated that soy protein intake is actually associated with a decreased risk of recurrence and a decreased risk of dying from breast cancer—even ER+ breast cancer. This decreased risk of cancer recurrence and death due to soy intake is evident in women receiving tamoxifen therapy, a known estrogen receptor–blocking agent, as well as in women not taking tamoxifen. The protective effect of soy is demonstrated in both menopausal and premenopausal women. The cancer-prevention effect of soy in women with a history of breast cancer was presented at the annual meeting of the American Association for Cancer Research in April 2011. Researcher Xiao Oh Shu, MD, analyzed four large epidemiological trials. After an average of nine years following their breast cancer diagnosis, women who ate more than 23 milligrams of soy per day (the equivalent of one glass of soy milk or one-half cup of tofu) lowered their risk of dying from any cause by 9 percent and reduced their risk for breast cancer recurrence by 15 percent compared to women who consumed 0.48 milligrams of soy per day or less.

Although the anticancer mechanism of soy is not fully understood, there are several well-evidenced theories. The isoflavones in soy slow the growth rate of cancer cells, have strong antioxidant effects, and reduce inflammation. Additionally, even though soy isoflavones bind to estrogen receptors, they preferentially bind to a certain type of estrogen receptor (estrogen receptor subtype beta) that seems to have an antigrowth effect. In summary, clinical trials indicate that soy consumption is associated with a decreased risk of cancers, including breast cancer, even in women with a history of ER+ breast cancer. Whole soy foods such as tofu, soy milk, edamame, and soy flour are associated with this preventive benefit. Isolated soy protein, found in snack bars or powders, lacks the beneficial isoflavones found in whole soy foods and because of this is not as beneficial. It is critical to choose organic sources of soy.

Q: *Can I drink any alcohol if I'm trying to prevent cancer?*

A: Many of us enjoy the pleasures of a glass of wine, a cocktail, or a beer. But drinking alcohol can be confusing to those with cancer, a history of cancer, or people trying to prevent cancer. Given the link between excess alcohol consumption and an increased risk of cancer, it's a valid concern.

In a prospective study of more than 350,000 adults, as part of the European Prospective Investigation into Cancer and Nutrition (EPIC) study published in the *British Medical Journal* in 2011, about 10 percent of all cancer in European men and 3 percent of all cancer in European women could be the result of current and former alcohol consumption. Cancers of the upper digestive tract (especially in men), liver cancer, and breast cancer in women are most attributable to alcohol intake. The majority of this risk is associated with moderate alcohol consumption, defined as more than two daily drinks for men or one daily drink for women. Greater than moderate alcohol consumption is causally related to cancers of the breast, colon, mouth, throat, esophagus, and liver, and the risk for all cancers increases with each additional daily drink. This means that there is a direct and linear relationship between the quantity of alcohol consumed over one's lifetime and the risk of cancer. In some situations, any alcohol consumption is problematic. For instance, in postmenopausal women who have a history of breast cancer, any regular alcohol consumption, of any type, increases the risk of breast cancer recurrence.

There is, however, an emerging body of research about the health benefits of moderate red wine consumption. Moderate consumption is defined as no more than 1 glass daily for women and up to 2 glasses daily for men. Red wine contains more than 20 different polyphenols, which are compounds that have potent antioxidant capacity, stimulate repair of damaged cells, reduce blood stickiness, stimulate the transport of cholesterol away from blood vessels to the liver for processing, reduce insulin resistance, and interrupt chronic inflammatory responses. Remember, polyphenols are powerful compounds. White wine only contains 10 percent of the polyphenols of red wine because the polyphenols are primarily derived from the dark pigmented compounds in grape skins. Interestingly, the greatest polyphenol content is found in red wine made from grapes exposed to significant sunlight and then macerated in oak barrels for the longest period of time. The oak tannins from the barrels add to the polyphenols, so red wine aged in oak barrels not only tastes good but is also healthier. According to the scientific literature, one daily glass of red wine reduces elevated blood sugar, is correlated with better weight control, and reduces inflammation— all of which are important cancer prevention strategies. This data would suggest that moderate alcohol consumption of the "right" alcohol may be more beneficial than harmful.

Q: Can I drink caffeinated beverages?

A: Some caffeinated beverages, such as coffee and tea, are not associated with increased cancer risk. In fact, coffee and tea are rich sources of polyphenols, contain powerful antioxidants, protect DNA, and have anti-inflammatory effects. Other caffeinated beverages, such as caffeinated soda, are not beneficial. Most soda pops have chemical additives and contain either lots of sugar or potentially cancer-causing sugar substitutes. Although caffeine is not, in and of itself, cancer-causing, drinking excess caffeine will compromise the stress response and, over time can contribute to excess cortisol. Elevated cortisol suppresses the immune system and is associated with increased inflammation and insulin resistance. Having one to two cups of coffee or black tea a day is unlikely to cause harm, and provides some protective effects.

Q: *Should I avoid dairy?*

A: Generally speaking, excessive reliance on dairy for calories, protein, or other nutrients is ill advised. Dairy is a source of saturated fat, and nonorganic dairy products contain residual antibiotics, hormones, and pesticides. Additionally, increased dairy consumption ups the risk of certain cancers, such as ovarian. On the flip side, dairy is a rich source of certain cancer-preventive compounds—namely conjugated linoleic acid (CLA) and vitamin K2. CLA has been demonstrated in several clinical studies to halt or slow the progression of tumors, as well as to increase cancer cell death. A 2011 meta-analysis (examination of several studies) showed that increased consumption of dairy food, but not milk, may actually be associated with a reduced risk of developing breast cancer. Dairy products, in particular butter (not to say we should be eating large amounts of butter), are rich sources of CLA. Vitamin K2 is an important vitamin in the control of angiogenesis, or the development of new blood vessels. As a tumor grows, it requires blood supply in order to keep growing. Inhibiting angiogenesis is a critical part of our internal defense against tumor growth. Dairy products, particularly cheese, are a rich source of vitamin K2. If you decide to include dairy in your diet, it is very important that it be organic. It is worth noting that the majority of vitamin K2 in our bodies is derived from the bacterial breakdown of foods in our digestive tract. Therefore, a good way to ensure adequate vitamin K2 is to make sure our digestive tracts contain sufficient beneficial bacteria. This can be accomplished by eating fermented foods such as yogurt (be sure it is natural, with low sugar content), sauerkraut, and kefir or taking a probiotic supplement every day.

Q: Do eggs contribute to an increased cancer risk?

A: The scientific data on the relationship between egg consumption and cancer risk is mixed. Some studies suggest that high intake of eggs is associated with an increased risk of certain cancers, namely ovarian, colon, and some other cancers of the digestive tract. However, other studies have failed to find this association. Until this association is further clarified, it may be appropriate to limit egg intake to less than seven eggs per week. It is also important to prepare eggs in a manner that avoids oxidizing their fats. The best methods of egg preparation are boiling and poaching. Frying and scrambling eggs denatures their cholesterol and fats, making them potentially deleterious to our health. Additionally, people at high risk for ovarian cancer and colon cancer should minimize egg intake. If you eat eggs, also purchase free-range, organic eggs.

Q: Does sugar feed cancer?

A: All the cells in the body rely on sugar to make energy, including cancer cells. Cancer cells are also very inefficient at metabolizing sugar into energy. As a result, cancer cells develop elaborate mechanisms to ensure they always have sufficient sugar supply. They even have increased insulin receptors on their surfaces so they can gobble up as much sugar as possible. In order for sugar to get inside a cell, it must have a chaperone, and that chaperone is insulin. When insulin binds to an insulin receptor on a cell membrane, the receptor changes shape, which allows sugar through the membrane and inside the cell. The numerous insulin receptors on cancer cells increase the likelihood that sugar will get in. So the short answer is that sugar does feed cancer; however, this is an oversimplification and misses the real dietary anticancer opportunity, which is connected to insulin resistance, one of our key five pathways.

In addition to shuttling sugar into cells, insulin also drives cell division and growth, which is not good when we are dealing with cancer cells. When insulin binds to an insulin receptor on the cancer cell, a message to divide is translated along a specific insulin-driven signaling pathway to the DNA of that cell. Insulin is a driver of cancer cell growth. When we consume a diet that consists primarily of simple carbohydrates and refined sugars, we are much more likely to develop insulin resistance. Insulin resistance is characterized by malfunctioning insulin receptors and a compensatory increase in blood levels of insulin. Because cancer cells have so many insulin receptors, even in an insulin-resistant state, cancer cells will still have enough receptors to bind insulin. Over time, excessive refined sugar consumption can increase insulin levels and "feed" the cancer. For this reason it is important to reduce one's consumption of simple sugars (e.g., refined sugar, candy, desserts, pastries). This does not mean reducing the intake of foods with naturally occurring sugar, such as fruits and vegetables. The thousands of cancer-fighting compounds that fruits and vegetables contain far outweigh the potential harm from their sugar. We should focus on the types of sugar we consume, avoiding simple sugars rather than fruits and vegetables.

Q: *Can I eat chocolate?*

A: Dark chocolate is a rich source of antioxidative and anti-inflammatory flavonoids. The flavonoids found in chocolate are similar to those found in green tea. The darker the chocolate—ideally at least 70 percent cocoa—the more flavonoids it contains. In fact, dark chocolate has twice the amount of flavonoids as does milk chocolate. Dark chocolate as a snack within a balanced diet has been demonstrated to improve DNA resistance to oxidative stress in humans for 22 hours. If you limit your consumption to quantities of two ounces or less, the sugar in the chocolate is unlikely to cause blood sugar issues. This is not true for pre-diabetics and diabetics, who should avoid chocolate sweetened with sugar. Organic dark chocolate that is minimally processed is the healthiest form of chocolate to eat. And remember, as described in the previous question, simple sugars other than those in dark chocolate should be avoided whenever possible.

Q: *Is the best cancer prevention diet a vegetarian diet?*

A: The best cancer prevention diet is a plant-based diet. Cancer prevention is associated with the consumption of five to 10 servings of vegetables every day. This does not, however, mean that you can't eat meat. As discussed previously, if you consume fish and/or lean meats from free-range, organically fed or grass-fed animals, you may obtain additional cancer prevention benefits. If you prefer to eat a vegetarian diet, there can be many health benefits. Vegetarians report higher energy levels, fewer weight problems, and general enhanced well-being. A healthy vegetarian diet should include five to 10 servings of vegetables a day and enough protein—typically 0.45 grams of protein per kilogram (2.2 pounds) of ideal body weight. That means that a 150-pound person should obtain a minimum of 30 grams of protein daily. If you are exercising daily, are pregnant, or have certain chronic diseases, your protein needs increase, often doubling or even tripling. Consuming sufficient protein while eating a vegetarian diet can be challenging and requires daily consumption of beans, legumes, tofu, and nuts.

Q: *Is it important to eat an alkaline diet?*

A: There are a variety of diets purported to have cancer-prevention effects due to the alkaline nature of the foods they are based upon. Generally, alkaline diets emphasize fresh and raw vegetables, nuts, and citrus fruits, while avoiding refined sugar, meat, dairy, and alcohol. According to advocates of the alkaline diet, the typical modern diet produces residual acid, particularly phosphates, which are acidic, after metabolism. Vegetarian diets, which tend to be alkaline, cause a person to have more alkaline urine than do diets containing high amounts of meat and dairy products. The idea behind an alkaline diet is that it assists the body's effort to maintain its acid/alkaline balance by supplying alkaline buffers. The theory holds that without alkaline buffers, the body will pull alkaline minerals from the bone, causing decreased bone density. However, several clinical trials have failed to demonstrate such a bone demineralization effect. These findings contradict the underlying rationale for alkaline diets, particularly given the fact that there are no clinical studies validating the dietary impact on alkaline/acid homeostasis.

Proponents of the alkaline diet assert that the residual acidity of the typical Western diet leads to tissue degeneration and chronic inflammatory diseases. While perhaps a compelling theory, there is no sound scientific evidence to support this contention. However, if following an alkaline diet means there is an increased focus on fruits and vegetables and a reduction of processed foods, we are all for it. Some alkaline diets, however, are extreme in nature and may not provide the balance required for long-term sustainability.

Q: *Do food allergies increase my risk of developing cancer?*

A: Food allergies are quite common, affecting as many as one in every three people. There is no proven link between consuming foods that create an immune-mediated allergic reaction (food allergens) and cancer. However, if an individual consumes food allergens repeatedly over months and years, there could be serious health consequences, including a predisposition to cancer development. Chronic consumption of food allergens impairs the health of all five key pathways. Food allergens can cause digestive distress that may lead to a leaky gut and imbalanced bacteria in the intestinal tract. It also creates chronic inflammation, which may manifest as joint pain, headaches, or sinusitis, among other ailments. Food allergies can also contribute to insulin resistance and disrupt sugar balance. Allergen consumption also favors humoral (antibody-driven) immunity over cytotoxic (direct cell-killing) immunity, which leads to autoimmune disease and impairs our cancer surveillance. Finally, eating allergens disrupts our hormones, including perpetuating high levels of the stress hormone cortisol, which, in turn, suppresses immune function. So, while a direct link between consuming food allergens and cancer has not been established in the scientific literature, there are multiple indirect links that are concerning. Determining whether you have food allergies is best done under the guidance of a naturopathic doctor or integrative healthcare practitioner who can administer an allergy elimination and challenge diet and/or order a blood test, such as the lymphocyte response assay/ELISA ACT test. These tests identify immune reactivity to a panel of foods, helping to determine which foods may be allergens.

Q: How worried should I be of bisphenol A (BPA) and other toxins found in food?

A: The bad news is that you should be very worried. The good news is that the detoxification system in the body helps us process these toxins. For more information about detoxification diets, refer to the sidebar on page 94). However, the detoxification system can get bogged down. The best way to reduce the amount of BPA in your diet is to reduce the amount of packaged and canned foods you eat. A 2011 study featured in the journal *Environmental Health Perspectives* demonstrated that both BPA and bis(2-Ethylhexyl) phthalate (DEHP) were substantially reduced when the study participants stuck with a fresh foods diet, versus foods that were canned and packed in plastic. This study actually showed a 66 percent reduction in BPA and upwards of a 56 percent reduction in DEHP in the urine of the study participants. Here are some other ways to reduce your exposure to toxins:

- Never microwave food in plastic containers.

- Avoid drinking out of aluminum cans.

- Look at the number on the bottom of plastic bottles:

  - Numbers 2, 4, and 5 are OK.

  - Number 1 should be used only one time and then discarded.

  - Numbers 3, 6, and 8 should be avoided.

- Reduce your exposure to secondhand smoke, and if you smoke, quit.

- Eat organic.

In this day and age, it's impossible to avoid all toxins in our food and environment. However, we can do things to reduce our exposure and support our internal detoxification pathway.

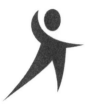 **HIGH FIVE TIP** *It may take time, but feeding your body what it needs is not complicated. In fact, diet is one thing our ancestors had right. Take time to cook your own food and to eat whole, unprocessed food. Follow your grandmother's footsteps into the kitchen to make eating enjoyable, flavorful, and fun. Appreciate the experience of eating, and you will appreciate the effects healthful food choices will have on your body.*

CHAPTER

DEEP **REJUVENATION**

E ven though you may be hoping to prevent a cancer diagnosis or recurrence, this is not adequate motivation to sustain you through the critical lifestyle changes. While the fear of the suffering, pain, expense, and ill health that cancer can bring can be initially motivating, these fears are not sufficient to keep us engaged in living a preventive lifestyle long term. It's not enough to simply want to prevent cancer. You need to want to live life with vitality.

The strongest sustaining factor is at the very core of our being. It is our desire to feel fully alive. This core sense of vitality is the most consistent and reliable way to stay engaged in those activities that bring us greater health. The purpose of prevention is to embrace living. This ability to rejoice in life is something that for many does not come easily. Sometimes, it even takes a diagnosis of cancer to give a person the opportunity to rediscover his most profound desire to be alive.

During the course of our work in integrative cancer care and education, we have had the honor and privilege of hearing many people's inspirational stories. JoAnne (not her real name), a 23-year-old woman with a diagnosis of advanced cervical cancer, is an intelligent, beautiful and studious individual. Prior to her diagnosis of cancer, she had battled throughout her teenage years with anorexia. With the diagnosis of her cancer, she wanted to learn as much as she could about the relationship between diet and cancer. As a result of her research, she determined that a macrobiotic diet (a diet that relies on grains and vegetables as the staple while avoiding processed or refined foods and most animal products) would be best for her.

Her mother, a caring and outspoken individual, was quite concerned about her daughter's dedication to a macrobiotic diet, given its restrictions and her daughter's history of anorexia. Despite her mother's concerns, JoAnne adopted a macrobiotic diet during her cancer treatment.

Over several months of treatment, JoAnne's already thin frame lost even more of its muscle mass. She began to look rather emaciated. Her mother became increasingly agitated, and when she accompanied her daughter to her chemotherapy treatments, she begged for help from anyone that would listen. One day, after hearing another round of her mother's pleas, something shifted in JoAnne's relationship to food. She asked herself this question, "Who are you feeding?" Something about the question made JoAnne pause. She considered this question deeply. Who was she feeding, or not feeding? As she thought about this question, she realized that her diet, healthy or not, was not feeding her. She had an epiphany as she realized that she was not even present in her body. In what seemed like an instant, she understood the act of eating as an act of nourishment, and in order to nourish oneself, one has to have a sense of being *worthy* of nourishment. With that awareness several other realizations came tumbling in.

For the first time in her life, JoAnne understood that she is an embodiment of life's energy. She finally had a deep appreciation for the precious nature of her life form and recognized her unique value and purpose. With this deepening awareness, she began to eat as a way to feed, nourish, and honor the life that she held. It was then that she realized her desire to truly live. She understood, really for the first time in her life, that she wanted to give this unique embodiment of life called JoAnne a chance to live with awareness and enthusiasm. This was really JoAnne's turning point in her care. Not only did she begin to respond to treatments, but she also emerged from this experience with a renewed sense of purpose and joy in living.

If we consider our life as a gift of enormous value, unique in all of creation, and of the most intricate design, then we are apt to care for this gift with reverence. Embarking upon a lifestyle that supports our health and vitality becomes more than a list of things to try to do better. All of a sudden, these diet changes, exercise programs, and dietary supplements become guideposts lighting our way toward complete immersion in the joy of living. It is this profound sense of joy that we hope to inspire. Even the title of our book reflects this perspective—it is Five to Thrive, not Five to Survive. For us, thriving is achieving a sense of no-holds-barred, full-on release into the joy and wonder of life. When this sense of exuberance permeates our being, we are compelled to live well. Exuberant living, even if felt as fleeting moments, is enough to sustain us on our path towards wellness. We deserve no less.

JOYFUL LIVING

Al Alschuler (Dr. Alschuler's father) was diagnosed with advanced pancreatic cancer in his early 60s. When he was diagnosed, he had just finished riding a hand-powered bicycle, "his Harley tricycle" as he would refer to it, from North Carolina to Massachusetts. For him, this trek was a spiritual odyssey, a way for him to better understand the limits of human endurance, the value of community, and the exhilaration of hard-won success. As he rode his way up the coast, he was also finishing a book on aging and on the process of dying. His diagnosis came just days after he finished both the ride and the first draft of his book. All of his exhilaration and sense of pride and accomplishment could have come crashing down when he received this diagnosis and its frighteningly dismal prognosis. Instead, true to his exuberant character, he decided to "greet Sister Death with [his] eyes wide open." Outliving his prognosis by more than a year, he lived each day of the next 17 months as if it were his last.

Now one might think that living each day as if it were your last would entail all forms of gluttony and immediate pleasures. Really though, living each day as if it is our last creates an acute sense of the value, the preciousness, and the wonder of life that is contained within each moment—an appreciation that transcends the material and stems from the heart. With this deep sense of appreciation, our desires become focused on gratitude and simply finding time to reflect on life. Al certainly had days of frustration, anger, and sadness, but he also spent an extraordinary number being deeply in love with life. This was, just as he had hoped, his greatest gift to not only his children but to all those who cared about him. In modeling the meaning of greeting death with his eyes wide open, he graciously showed those he loved the meaning of living life fully and exuberantly.

Short of facing impending death or witnessing the death of a loved one, there are many ways we can discover this deep sense of joyful living. For example, in the middle of a busy day, find a comfortable seat near a window where the early afternoon sunshine is streaming in and simply close your eyes and let yourself feel the warmth and coziness of the sun's rays. Soak in the deep sense of peaceful contentedness in that moment. You can also experience this profound sense of gratitude for life by inhaling that first aroma of freshly brewed coffee in the morning and cherishing the anticipation of the first sip. Reaching out for a loved one's hand and clasping it in yours is another simple yet profound connection to life. It is these brief moments that both remind us and allow us to experience the deeply rooted ecstasy of life. These are the moments we truly live for. Pausing and recognizing the frequency of these moments and then artfully stringing them together helps us create our joyful living landscape.

Eating a healthy diet, exercising every day, and taking all the right supplements may prevent cancer. However, these actions in the absence of a profound sense of the value of life will not grant us sustainable and joyful health and vitality. Health is, after all, more than the mere absence of disease. We advocate a program of health and prevention that is interwoven with a renewed love of life and desire to embrace our being completely.

SURRENDER

You may think of "surrender" as giving up or showing weakness; however, we like to think of it as a sign of strength and letting go. In many ways, our ability to embrace life requires surrender. For some, the surrender comes moments before they die. These

SURRENDERING WITH SERENITY

By Dr. Alschuler

One person that personifies this lesson is Barbara (not her real name), a who was diagnosed with advanced bladder cancer in her 50s. Barbara had led a difficult life. She had a permanent dour expression etched on her face, and only spoke in short, clipped sentences. She seemed as if life was something she just had to put up with, and she certainly didn't appear to be having any fun. Despite years of treatment, the cancer ultimately spread throughout her body.

I met with Barbara throughout her chemotherapy and every time I saw her I inquired about her health and offered suggestions about various supportive therapies. Sometimes Barbara would agree, but most of the time she declined. One day, I learned that Barbara had been admitted to the hospital. Her liver had begun to fail and she only had a matter of days left to live. I immediately went to see her. I went to Barbara's side and grasped her hand. She returned the grasp with surprising strength. Barbara whispered, "Please don't let go". For a while, I simply sat on the edge of Barbara's bed holding her hand. I then turned to her and saw a tear escaping down the side of her cheek. I asked her if there was anything I could do for her. Barbara whispered back, "Home, I miss home." I remembered that Barbara had told me that her home was in the country and she had mentioned a pond in the back of her house. I started to speak to Barbara about the pond so she could imagine it. I described the changes a pond goes through throughout the seasons. I described a flock of geese that discovered the pond and the sound of their wings hitting the water as they flapped their way somewhere else for the winter. I described everything I could think of related to this serene spot of nature. As I spoke, her hand lessened its grip and her breathing became less labored and her face took on a less strained expression.

Many hours later and well into the evening, I left the now sleeping Barbara. The next morning, I learned that Barbara had died shortly after I left her room. I was surprised by my sense of loss given how challenging a patient Barbara had been. But then I realized that I had shared a very profound moment with Barbara. She had finally allowed herself to experience peace, connection, and comfort—and this was how she died. In so doing, Barbara imparted a tremendous gift by allowing me to love her unconditionally, offer complete forgiveness, and connect with another being around the simple and graceful beauty of life manifested in nature. These fundamental attributes – unconditional love, complete forgiveness, and awe – are exactly those required to rejuvenate our life's purpose. Our job is to surrender ourselves to this possibility.

individuals are fortunate to experience a sense of peace as their last sensation before dying, and they undoubtedly would wish they had experienced this sense of peace along their journey rather than only at the end. Throughout our work in the field of cancer care, we have had the opportunity to spend time with people in the end stages of cancer. Many of these experiences have been incredible gifts and have taught us the lesson of the sacredness of life over and over again. These stories have also illustrated and emphasized the importance of surrender. For more information on surrender, refer to the story on the previous page.

THE FIVE Rs

We ultimately require no instruction on how to surrender into love, forgiveness, or living life in awe. However, there are some strategies that make it easier to bring these attributes into our daily lives. These strategies form the foundation of our rejuvenation plan toward thriving. Here are our five Rs to rejuvenation:

1. Rhythm
2. Rest
3. Relaxation
4. Replenishment
5. Rehydration

Each of these concepts helps to facilitate our ability to experience our lives fully and completely. These Five Rs create a significant sense of wellness on a psychological/emotional/spiritual level, but also on the physical plane as well. In fact, these five Rs are powerful epigenetic change agents that optimize the health of each of our five key bodily pathways. Let's delve a little deeper into each one.

RHYTHM

In large part, our bodies function in accordance with built-in rhythms that are dictated by the natural world around us. These are called circadian rhythms, and they influence our bodily functions in a patterned way each day. These daily rhythms are driven by an internal clock, which responds to the change from day to night. The central clock of this bodily timekeeping system is located in the brain and is synchronized to daylight through photoreceptors in the eyes. Time related messages are sent out as hormones and as electrical signals that travel along our nerves. These hormonal and nerve messages sync secondary clocks found within the cells of our organs to our central clock. In this way, the body's actions keep rhythm with the world around us.

The most obvious example of circadian rhythms is our natural wakefulness during the day and sleepiness at night. This is due, in part, to the nighttime stimulation of melatonin. Melatonin is a hormone secreted by the pineal gland in the brain. Melatonin causes us to feel sleepy and suppresses the activity of many cellular functions, enabling our bodies to rest. Our wakefulness during the day begins as our eyes are exposed to morning light. This triggers a shutdown of melatonin production. At the same time, early in the morning, the level of certain wakefulness hormones, such as cortisol from the adrenal gland, rises. Cortisol follows a daily pattern, reaching its highest level in the morning and lowest in the evening.

Many other bodily functions, including the five key pathways that we emphasize, are under the influence of our internal clocks, so creating a natural rhythm is important to optimize their functioning. Fat metabolism and insulin secretion are influenced by our circadian rhythm and fluctuate throughout the day. The activity of our immune cells is under circadian influence as well.

This rhythmic influence is so strong that if we become disconnected from our innate clock—for instance if we work the night shift or stay up into the early hours of the morning and then sleep during the day—our immune cells are much less efficient at recognizing threats and destroying invaders. Altered circadian rhythms also reduce our resistance to environmental stressors, accelerating oxidative and inflammatory damage. People with impaired circadian rhythms develop digestive insufficiency, may experience constipation or diarrhea, and may develop changes in the bacterial balance in the digestive tract.

Disrupting our circadian rhythm by becoming out of sync with the normal cycle of day and night will over time impair each of the five key bodily pathways:

- The immune system will not function efficiently.

- We will develop chronic inflammation.

- Hormonal cycles will become unbalanced—particularly the hypothalamic-pituitary-adrenal (HPA) axis, which controls stress response via cortisol production.

- We may develop insulin resistance.

- Our ability to digest foods and detoxify toxins will become compromised.

The net long-term result of this disarray can be chronic disease, including cancer. Thus, the health impact of regaining normal circadian rhythms cannot be overstated.

For most of us this is as simple as retraining ourselves to go to sleep soon after it becomes dark and to wake with the beginning of daylight. The artificial lights we have in our modern society have enabled us to experience very long days and short nights. This pattern of living is at odds with our internal clocks. While it may not be possible to go to bed at eight every night and wake up at six in the morning, it should be possible for most people to adjust their schedules to facilitate more sleep when it's dark and more activity when it's light. Even after several weeks of this schedule, one's circadian rhythm will regain its synchronicity, and with this, health will improve.

If you have a schedule that is out of sync with your internal clock, it is typically helpful to make adjustments in small increments. If your bedtime is too late, start going to bed five minutes earlier. Bump your bedtime back five minutes every week until you reach your target. The importance of establishing consistent rhythms is vital and well worth the retraining effort. Although deviations from your normal schedule will happen from time to time, the occasional late night will not unravel the health benefits that you have gained as long as most of your days are lived in the right rhythm—activity in daylight and sleeping at nighttime.

REST

We should get eight hours of sleep each night, yet more than one-third of Americans sleep only six hours or less. Furthermore, some people who get sufficient hours of sleep are not getting high-quality sleep. The 2002 National Sleep Foundation Sleep in America poll found that approximately 15 percent of people in the United States suffer from a sleep disorder. The most common sleep disorder is insomnia, defined as difficulty falling asleep, frequent nighttime waking, and not feeling refreshed in the morning. The link between lack of sleep and poor health is getting stronger. Insufficient sleep—either in amount or quality—impacts each of our five key bodily pathways. Here's how.

Immune: The impact of sleep deprivation on immune function is complex. With a few nights of poor sleep, there is often a transitory increase in the activity of some of our immune cells. However, if prolonged, immune function will become suppressed and imbalanced. Cytotoxic immunity, the direct cell-killing component of immune function, is the most sensitive to sleep deprivation. As our primary defense against cancer, decreased cytotoxic immunity from sleep deprivation increases our risk of cancer.

Inflammation: Many clinical studies on the effects of sleep loss in humans have shown that chronic inflammation increases in sleep-deprived individuals. For example, individuals who "pull an all-nighter" have elevated levels of inflammatory cytokines. Inflammatory markers are also elevated in people who only sleep four to six hours a night. A clinical study involving healthy men found that after a night of sleep deprivation (they were only allowed to sleep for two hours), various inflammatory markers, including cortisol, increased. In subjects who recovered by taking a nap followed by an eight-hour sleep and in individuals who recovered by an extended sleep (10 hours), all inflammatory markers returned to normal. This is good news, because it suggests that we can rebalance the inflammatory effects of sleep deprivation with extra sleep.

Hormones: Sleep disruption acts as a stressor to the body and, as such, activates the HPA axis. This axis is our primary stress response system, and when it's activated it kicks various stress hormones (e.g., cortisol, IL-6) into gear. Chronically sleep-deprived people do not have the opportunity to reset their HPA axis. Over time, these people will develop chronically elevated stress hormones, which can cripple immune function, unravel digestion, increase anxiety and depression, impede memory, impair blood sugar control, delay wound healing, and raise blood pressure. As you can see, if our HPA axis cannot reset, we will experience profound negative impacts on our health. Sleep deprivation also alters thyroid hormone levels, estrogen and testosterone secretion, and many other hormones involved in regulating cellular activity and growth. Both the amount and the secretion pattern of hormones are affected by sleep deprivation. Disrupted patterns of hormonal secretion can be as damaging to our health.

Insulin Resistance: Several studies have demonstrated that lack of sleep increases insulin resistance, which is a risk factor for many illnesses including diabetes and cancer. In 2011, a study featured in *Clinical Endocrinology & Metabolism* demonstrated that even just one night of partial sleep deprivation (four hours or less) induced signs of insulin resistance. Years of short sleep (defined as sleeping less than six hours) induces insulin resistance and is associated with obesity and diabetes. When we are sleep-deprived, we disrupt the daily circadian rhythm that controls blood sugar balance, and we can lose insulin sensitivity. Our bodies are simply not programmed to manage our blood sugar levels on insufficient sleep.

Digestion and Detoxification: During sleep when no thought is required, our autonomic nervous system, which controls the activity of our glands and organs, is dominated by parasympathetic nerve activity. Parasympathetic activity slows down heart rate, increases digestive activity, and stimulates urination and sexual function. The balancing part of our autonomic nervous system, sympathetic activity, is often referred to as our fight-or-flight response. It speeds up heart rate, dilates pupils, opens blood vessels allowing more blood to get to muscles, and increases breathing. If we are sleep-deprived, we have increased sympathetic activity and decreased parasympathetic activity. One result of this state is that the digestive system does not receive sufficient stimulation. Over time, this will compromise the regularity of bowel movements, which, in turn, will affect the type and quantity of bacteria in our intestines. Imbalanced bacteria and altered bowel regularity will disrupt the integrity of our intestines— possibly leading to leaky gut syndrome, which facilitates the absorption of toxins from the intestines into our blood. These toxins require detoxification by the liver, and if copious amounts are released it can overwhelm the liver detoxification pathway. When this happens, our cells are left vulnerable to carcinogens that are normally detoxified. Thus, in an insidious manner, sleep deprivation harms our digestion and detoxification pathway and increases our risk for cancer.

BOTTOM LINE ABOUT SLEEP

Sufficient sleep is a must. Unfortunately, there are many factors that can interfere with the quality of our sleep. These include unresolved stress, a noisy environment, too much light in the bedroom, hormonal issues such as hot flashes, too much alcohol, insufficient protein in the evening meal, and side effects from medications. If you are having trouble getting a good night's rest, it is important to survey your life to see what might be causing the trouble. In addition to these issues, here are some tips to getting a good night's rest:

- Keep your bedroom dark and quiet.

- Exercise daily to prevent pent-up energy from keeping you awake.

- Eat protein at dinnertime so your blood sugar remains better balanced over the night; some people experience poor sleep because drops in blood sugar awaken them.

- Consider taking a dietary supplement such as L-theanine (Suntheanine®), valerian, chamomile, 5-HTP, homeopathic remedies, or melatonin.

It is best to seek advice from a qualified healthcare practitioner before starting on these supplements to avoid any interactions with other medications or other unintended side effects. If you are experiencing difficulties with sleep, talk to a healthcare professional about your options. Getting the proper amount of rest each day is absolutely critical to your health.

RELAXATION

The third R is relaxation. Relaxation is different from rest but is just as essential to rejuvenating our health. Rest is tied more directly to the physical act of sleeping and resting, while relaxation is a state of well-being. In many ways, relaxation is the opposite of stress. When we allow ourselves to feel relaxed, we let go of feelings of stress, anxiety, and depression. By allowing ourselves to experience deep, consistent relaxation, we facilitate our body's ability to regain internal homeostasis (balance). Relaxation also serves the critical role of creating the time and space needed to restore our mental and emotional balance. Unfortunately, the pace of modern living is somewhat antithetical to relaxation. Most of us are working long hours, perhaps raising a family, and usually multitasking. We are constantly calling upon ourselves to do more.

A classic example of someone in this category is a caregiver. Caregivers have some of the highest stress levels of any group of people. Research has shown that caregivers have increased gene expression of pro-inflammatory genes, namely NF-kappaB, C-reactive protein and IL-1. The constant and severe stress of caregiving epigenetically influences genes that make inflammatory compounds. When these genes are activated to produce these compounds, the risk for inflammatory diseases such as cancer and heart disease increases. Stress reduction is critical to all of us but is especially important for caregivers.

One of the most prevalent stresses that people experience is anxiety. Many people have some level of anxiety most of the time. Research has shown that anxiety is actually a manifestation of our body's defense against stress. When we encounter stress, our HPA axis responds to the stress by secreting cortisol, epinephrine, and interleukins. These chemicals influence many other key bodily functions as we have discussed previously.

Another effect of these compounds is to alter brain activity and neurotransmitter production in a way that favors a state of anxiety. This makes sense if you think about the fact that when we encounter stress, it's natural for us to feel anxious in order to create discomfort, which in turn motivates us to move away from the stress. However, experiencing chronic anxiety can be very disruptive to overall health. People who are anxious tend to eat poorly, don't exercise, and can't sleep well. Anxious people also tend to drink more alcohol. None of these behaviors is conducive to healthful living. Not to mention the fact that chronic anxiety is itself a form of distress. If unresolved, this distress will create a generalized sense of loss of control. Once this state of being is reached, it is very difficult to summon the inner resources necessary to proactively engage in a healthy preventive lifestyle. In fact, one of the most important messages of the Five to Thrive anticancer plan is one of empowerment. Feeling empowered to make and sustain healthful changes is a necessary ingredient to long-term success and is healing in and of itself.

Relaxation is the antidote to anxiety. The path to relaxation is different for each person. Whether it comes from taking a walk in the woods, playing a musical instrument, spending time with a friend over a cup of tea, receiving a therapeutic massage, or meditating, the end result will be the same. The most important thing is to figure out what relaxes you and then to prioritize that activity so you experience relaxation *every day*. Make a list of five things that help you relax, and then make a commitment to do one of those five things every day. Before you begin your day, ask yourself "How am I going to relax today?" and then schedule that relaxing activity just as you would an important meeting.

In our type-A society, relaxation and downtime can be frowned upon. People who are not busy all of the time may be seen as unproductive loafers. Nothing could be further from the truth. People who engage in regular relaxation are actively building their health. Health does not happen in the background of our lives; it requires a diverse mix of ingredients, including relaxation. It's time to shed any guilt and step confidently into a life that includes regular relaxing downtime.

REPLENISH

The fourth R is for replenish. On one level, replenishment means simply supplying of nutrients to the body to meet its needs for optimal functioning. The chapters on diet and dietary supplements describe the essential nutrients for a comprehensive cancer prevention plan. Nutrition is so critical that we devoted an entire chapter to the subject. In this section, replenishment takes on additional meaning. In order to rejuvenate one's sense of health and well-being, we must replenish the components of life that have been left unattended and neglected. There is not a magic formula that works for everyone, but certain aspects of life require replenishment in order to sustain most of us.

In addition to replenishing our physical bodies with food, sleep, and movement, our spirit needs replenishing as well. One of the things we have been most struck by while meeting people across the country affected by cancer is how depleted many of them feel. It is almost as if cancer entered their lives and robbed them of all of their emotional reserves. Studies have shown that feelings of fatigue and exhaustion after successful cancer treatment are common. Up to one-third of breast cancer survivors experience persistent fatigue, which has been linked to a heightened state of stress and nervous system overdrive. This state causes the release of inflammatory chemicals that further contribute to the fatigue. This vicious cycle takes these survivors about as far from replenishment as they can get. Sadly, even if they recover their energy and zest for life once treatment is over, many people experience worry and anxiety about cancer recurrence.

THE NEEDLE KNOWS

Acupuncture is a procedure that involves stimulation of the body's energy known as qi (pronounced chee). It is primarily used to treat a variety of conditions, but it can also be used to balance and replenish the body and even to help reduce stress and anxiety. The National Institutes of Health (NIH) consensus statement explains that acupuncture has demonstrated promising results for a variety of conditions including pain, nausea, asthma and others. The NIH concludes, "Further research is likely to uncover additional areas where acupuncture interventions will be useful." We are not only strong advocates of acupuncture we have both experienced positive personal results from it. Be sure to consult with an acupuncturist who is properly licensed, comes with a strong referral, and is trained in this unique and effective form of medicine.

This further zaps their emotional resilience and can leave them feeling chronically burned out. In some of these people a new cancer prevention plan can become yet another burden. Even if the precepts of the plan are healthful, the net effect can be harmful. For this reason, replenishment of one's emotional and spiritual reserve is critical to long-term prevention and a healthy life—not just for those trying to prevent a recurrence, but for everyone trying to prevent cancer. Although many ways exist to replenish emotional and spiritual vitality, a few are universally beneficial.

One of the most important ways to replenish our vitality is through laughter and love. In fact, when we give our presentation on integrative cancer care, despite the serious nature of the topic, we always include jokes, lighthearted teasing, and humor in these presentations. We do this because we want each presentation to replenish the spirits of those in attendance as well as our own. One of the most gratifying experiences for us is to watch people, many of whom are quite ill, laugh and smile throughout our presentation. We know that a laughing person's soul is being replenished. That's why this book includes an entire chapter on love, laughter, and joy.

Expressing ourselves creatively is also a particularly effective way to replenish ourselves. Several studies have shown that being creative benefits the elderly by improving mood, boosting self-esteem, and encouraging socialization. According to a 2008 *Washington Post* exposé, several well-designed studies have shown that creative activity causes physiological changes that increase brain function, as well as the expression of joy.

We may think of creativity as art or acting, but it's so much more. Being creative can entail visiting museums, craft stores, or local boutiques. It can include journaling, doing puzzles, or joining a book club. Being creative means that you agree to put rules aside. You are coloring outside the lines. Whatever you create is just that—something you create. You don't have to produce masterpieces and you can discard anything that you make; the replenishment comes from the doing. Just by being open to your own creativity and to that characteristic in others, you will feel replenished and experience a renewed sense of playfulness.

Speaking of being playful, that's still another way to replenish and recharge your inner spark. A young man came up to us after one of our talks and told us about how he had started running in his nearby park. He was so pleased as his distance increased until he was finally able to run several miles through the park to a swing set on the other side. As a reward, he frequently ended his run with a swing on the swings. "At first I thought I must look silly, a grown man swinging on the swings, but then I realized I didn't care. I felt like a kid again." Sometimes we can achieve replenishment in unsuspecting ways, and being playful can be one of the most joyous ways to do that. And the best part of being playful is that it often involves smiling, laughing, and loving—key ingredients to replenishment success!

REHYDRATION

The average human body is 60 percent water. Water is critical to life. It is so important and yet so simple that it just doesn't get emphasized enough. That is why we have included rehydration as our fifth R. Here are just some of the key ways water functions in the body:

- It is used to make blood.
- The cerebrospinal fluid that nourishes the brain and nerves requires water.
- The fluid that cushions our joints is made from water.
- Water contributes to digestive juices and bile, which helps us absorb fat.
- It is added to digestive waste products so they can be eliminated.
- It helps maintain our body temperature.
- It nourishes our cells.

Just how much water does the body need for all these important jobs? A common recommendation is to drink eight cups of water each day, in order to replace what most people naturally lose (about eight to nine cups of water) each day through sweat, urination, and breathing. Rehydrating ourselves with eight cups of water daily will help us to preserve enough water to maintain essential functions. Another good way to ingest water is to consume foods with high water content. These include most fruits and vegetables. On the flip side, coffee and alcohol are dehydrating. Thus minimizing their consumption or at the very least adding extra water to compensate for their dehydrating effect is important. It is also important to drink extra water after you exercise, as exercise depletes extra water through sweat and increased respiration.

When drinking water, it is important to drink high-quality water. Water that has been filtered through reverse osmosis and/or carbon filtration is ideal, as filtration removes significant quantities of cancer-causing compounds from the water. Water that is more alkaline may be more beneficial than acidic water in that alkaline water is associated in some clinical studies with decreased bone loss. Adequate bone density is an important aspect of long-term wellness.

Drink water from a glass, ceramic, or stainless steel container. Plastic water bottles, although convenient, contain hormonally active compounds called bisphenols. These compounds can be toxic and disrupt hormonal balance. The thickness and type of plastic will determine the level of exposure to bisphenols. It's worth repeating that the numbers on the bottom of plastic are important. Remember:

- Numbers 3, 6, and 7 should be avoided
- Number 1 should be a one-time use only
- Numbers 2, 4, and 5 are OK to use

Hard to remember? Try our pneumonic: "2, 4, and 5 will keep me alive but 3, 6, and 7 may send me to heaven."

Drink water as your main beverage. It is alright to flavor water with a small amount of juice, freshly squeezed citrus, or herbal teas. If you are struggling to consume enough water, try drinking it with a straw, varying its flavor, and drinking water before every meal. As you increase your water intake, you will soon become thirsty if you drop your consumption—so it really does get easier as you go.

IN CONCLUSION

Rejuvenation is about rediscovering our love of life. Within this joyful embrace resides the foundation of health and vitality. Rejuvenation is fundamental to cancer prevention and to overall health. Rejuvenation requires getting back to the basics with the foundational five Rs: rhythm, rest, relaxation, replenishment, and rehydration. From there, the vitality and sacredness of our lives will bloom into every day.

 **HIGH FIVE TIP** *Words often used to describe rejuvenation include vigor, restoration, and freshness—all feelings we long to have. One way to help us gain these feelings is to evaluate how you feel with a large group of people. Are you recharged by such interactions or do you find that you become drained if you are around people all the time? Perhaps you are an introvert, or at least require some introversion to recharge your battery. Being in touch with what you need to recharge is critical, and it just may mean that sometimes you need to be alone.*

CHAPTER 7

PROD THE PATHWAYS WITH
DIETARY SUPPLEMENTS

We like to think of dietary supplements as prongs of a pitchfork. Precisely chiseled, these prongs are able to fit into the nooks and crannies of our biochemical pathways to leverage their power. Dietary supplements can create precise epigenetic changes in the health of our key pathways by influencing our internal landscape on a cellular level.

Dietary supplements are an area of emphasis during our presentations. Invariably, nearly all of the questions during the Q&A involve dietary supplement use. "There are so many choices," lament our audience participants. "Where do I even begin?" While it's true that countless dietary supplements could benefit our health and have significant cancer prevention actions, taking dozens of supplements every day may not be feasible physically or financially. We remind our audience members, "Dietary supplements are called supplements for a reason: They are meant to supplement the diet and should not be used as replacements for healthy eating." The role of dietary supplements are to augment a healthy diet and lifestyle by providing additional, targeted molecular support. And that's what this chapter is all about. It's also about helping you prioritize which dietary supplements to take.

Following is an overview of what we consider to be foundational dietary supplements beneficial for most people. We have selected the supplements that have the biggest potential to improve health and help prevent cancer. The supplements we discuss are backed by scientific research and clinical experience. They were chosen because they influence all five pathways. Remember, when we effectively support all five pathways, we can change the epigenetic influences on our cells. Over time, this gentle yet precise impact can radically alter the terrain in the body and create an environment that disfavors cancer development.

Our dietary supplement foundation consists of five groups of dietary supplements with both short- and long-term benefits on our health, as well as significant cancer prevention actions:

1. Omega-3 fatty acids

2. Probiotics

3. Polyphenols

4. Antioxidants

5. Vitamin D

Let's take a closer look at all five.

OMEGA-3 FATTY ACIDS

Omega-3 fatty acids are part of a larger group of fats called essential fatty acids. In the body, omega-3 fatty acids are derived from alpha-linolenic acid (ALA). From ALA, the body makes all other omega-3 fatty acids, including eicosapentaenoic acid (EPA) and docosahexaenoic acid (DHA). Some individuals, however, cannot convert ALA into EPA or DHA because they lack sufficient activity of a critical enzyme needed for this conversion. This metabolic challenge, combined with the fact that most people don't ingest large enough quantities of ALA, has led to a population-wide deficiency in omega-3 fatty acids. That's one reason why omega-3 is a foundational nutritional supplement in our program.

Omega-3 fatty acids are found in fish, fish oils, vegetables, nuts, and seeds. Vegetable oils lack EPA and DHA but do have ALA. Non-hydrogenated canola oil, flaxseeds, walnuts, and other nuts and seeds are rich sources of ALA. The typical North American diet includes about 1 to 3 grams of ALA each day. However, the typical North American diet lacks EPA and DHA, providing only 0.10 to 0.15 grams per day. Additionally, this diet contains high amounts— as much as 12 to 15 grams—of omega-6 fatty acids such as lin-

DIETARY SUPPLEMENT POPULARITY CONTINUES TO SOAR

In a study conducted by the Centers for Disease Control and Prevention (CDC) in 2011, more than one-half of U.S. adults said they take dietary supplements. This result was based on data collected from surveying adults between the years of 2003 and 2006 and comparing it to data collected in 1988 to 1994. Not only did more than half of all Americans take supplements, but the percentage increased since 1994. Another survey conducted by the National Center for Health Statistics found that in 2007, more than 40 percent of American adults used complementary and alternative medicine, most including dietary supplements. While billions of Americans take dietary supplements, over half do not disclose this use to their doctors. Because supplements can interact with medications, you should always inform all of your healthcare providers about your supplement usage.

oleic acid. That means that most people have an overabundance of omega-6 with deficiencies in omega-3 fatty acids—particularly EPA and DHA. The ratio of omega-6 to omega-3 fatty acids is as important as an overt deficiency of the omega-3 fatty acids. This imbalanced ratio predisposes the body to inflammation, alters immune function, increases insulin resistance, and increases cellular susceptibility to damage. And, as you might suspect, omega-3 fatty acids positively influence all five key pathways!

The most dramatic impact of omega-3 fatty acids—particularly EPA and DHA—is on the inflammatory pathway. Omega-3 fatty acids influence cellular membranes and change critical cell-signaling mechanisms. As a result, omega-3 fatty acids can alter gene expression and influence key cellular processes. The net result of these influences is reduced production of inflammatory cytokines, the chemicals that stimulate inflammation in our bodies. This anti-inflammatory effect from EPA and DHA is why fish oils have received so much attention for the prevention of heart disease. These same anti-inflammatory effects have been demonstrated in cancer prevention as well. High intake of EPA and DHA reduces many of the inflammatory molecules (things like C reactive protein, interleukin-6 and homocysteine) that are elevated in people with aggressive cancers.

Omega-3 fatty acids also increase insulin sensitivity and help normalize blood sugar levels. Even in obese, insulin resistant

THE RELUCTANT PILL POPPER
GOES SHOPPING By Dr. Alschuler

Joe (not his real name) did not have it easy. After being treated for colon cancer, he was cancer-free but was left with the unfortunate side effect of severe diarrhea. He had little control of his bowels and could only leave his house safely for a couple of hours at a time. He came to see me and declared, "I want to have my life back, but I don't want to take any pills."

Over the next couple of months, Joe adopted significant dietary changes that I suggested and his diarrhea became a little more manageable. Unfortunately, he still couldn't trust himself to be far from a bathroom for more than a few hours. I finally said to Joe that if he would be willing to try some pills for one month, I thought I could help him. When the month was up, I promised, he could decide whether to continue. I carefully selected my supplement recommendations, and he left with three different supplements that each required taking several capsules each day.

A month went by, and Joe came back in to see me. He was wearing an impressive black cowboy hat that I had never seen before. I commented on the hat. He took it off his head and turned it over and pointed out the special features of this hat. He then said, "This hat was hard to find. I had to look for a while. In fact, I was out shopping for this hat for five hours." He looked up and smiled, "I guess I should have bought some new pants too, seeing as how I will be needing deeper pockets to carry my pills around with me." We both laughed.

I think about Joe when I hear from people who have never taken supplements or don't think they can or want to take supplements. Taking pills is not for everyone, but even the biggest naysayer may encounter something in his life that inspires in him a desire to use supplements. And, when that happens, it will be important to be armed with the knowledge and resources.

adults, a diet high in cod increases insulin sensitivity. Interestingly, one of the mechanisms of this increased insulin sensitivity from cod may be due to a reduction in inflammation, specifically high-sensitivity C reactive protein.

Omega-3 fatty acids support immunity by increasing macrophage function. Macrophages are immune cells that are like roving eyes that recognize a cancerous cell and then alert the rest of the immune system to destroy it. Here is where the ratio of fatty acids comes into play. Individuals with high omega-6 and low omega-3 tend to be immunosuppressed. As the ratio changes from an increased intake of EPA and DHA, immune function increases. This has even been demonstrated in patients who are undergoing major surgery. Those who receive added omega-3 fatty acids to their nutritional supplementation after surgery have reduced risk of infection and sepsis (a very serious, life-threatening bloodborne infection).

Omega-3 fatty acids have an interesting relationship to detoxification. One of the key enzymes that the liver uses to detoxify compounds is called glutathione-S-transferase. In addition to metabolizing toxins, glutathione-S-transferase also breaks down the metabolic byproducts of omega-3 fats. As the body uses omega-3 fats, a process known as lipid peroxidation occurs and generates peroxide metabolites that are toxic to our cells. Glutathione-S-transferase binds to these toxins and eliminates them. Research shows that women who have genetically or epigenetically decreased activity of glutathione-S-transferase enzyme activity and cannot get rid of these peroxides very efficiently also experience a significantly higher than normal cancer-preventive effect from omega-3 fatty acids. In fact, high intake of omega-3 fatty acids appears to cut breast cancer risk by up to 74 percent in women with low glutathione-S-transferase activity. Omega-3 fatty acids generate compounds that are directly toxic to cancer cells. This effect was put to the test in an animal study on omega-3 and omega-6 fatty acids in response to tamoxifen. Researchers from the University of Texas Health and Science Center found that a diet rich in omega-3 fatty acids along with tamoxifen had nearly 80 percent tumor growth inhibition demonstrating a synergistic effect, possibly by generating peroxides.

Ingestion of omega-3 fatty acids has been linked with decreased risk of a variety of cancers in clinical trials. People at high risk for colon cancer treated with omega-3 fatty acids for 30 days had decreased tumor cell proliferation, as well as decreased inflammatory activity. Supplemental omega-3 fatty acids have also been shown to reduce the pro-inflammatory and immunosuppressive reaction to ultraviolet radiation in human skin, thereby reducing risk for non-melanoma skin cancer. Omega-3 fatty acids from flaxseed have been demonstrated to inhibit breast cancer cell growth and exert anti-estrogen effects. This seems to be the result of both the essential fatty acids and other compounds in flaxseed known as lignans. There is also evidence that omega-3 ingestion can help prevent prostate cancer growth because of its anti-inflammatory effects; however, the scientific evidence for omega-3s and prostate cancer prevention is mixed. Researchers from the Fred Hutchinson Cancer Research Center in Seattle found that men with the highest blood percentages of DHA had two-and-a-half-times the risk of developing aggressive, high-grade prostate cancer compared to men with the lowest DHA levels. Of note, most of the men obtained these high levels from eating fish. Fish can be, unfortunately, a common source of heavy metals and other pollutants that are independently linked with cancer risk.

It can be difficult to consume enough omega-3 fatty acids every day to get the anticancer benefits, but a variety of EPA and DHA supplements are available. The most important factor when choosing an EPA and DHA supplement is to evaluate the quality of the supplement, particularly for those oils extracted from fish. Many forms of marine life are now contaminated with high levels of heavy metals such as mercury, and these metals can show up in supplements. Furthermore, the extraction process of EPA and DHA can be done with a bleaching process that utilizes dioxin, a cancer-causing substance. If this dioxin is not removed from the final product, it will be present in the fish oil supplements.

Another important parameter of fish oil quality involves freshness. Fish oil that has been poorly extracted can become rancid. These products tend to have a strong fishy odor, and their health benefits are questionable. When purchasing an EPA and DHA supplement, look for a third-party certification quality seal on the label. It is worth the time to contact the manufacturer and ask them about their manufacturing process and ask for a copy of their certificate of analysis for the lot of product that you have purchased. This certificate of analysis should demonstrate that the product has been tested for, and is absent of, heavy metals, dioxins, and rancidity. Some companies post these certificates of analyses on their website. Integrative healthcare practitioners can also guide you to the best quality fish oil supplements.

A unique product called Vectomega offers a high quality option. Researchers studying absorption of omega 3 fatty acids have found that EPA and DHA that are bound to phospholipids absorb up to 50 times better than standard fish oil. Vectomega is a phospholipid-based extract of salmon that was developed by scientists at the University of Nancy, in France. Because of its absorption, you only need to take one or two tablets a day to meet your omega 3 needs. This product is distributed exclusively in the U.S. by EuroPharma, Inc., in their Terry Naturally line of supplements. For people who prefer fish oil-based supplements, we also suggest Kyolic-EPA®, which contains the proper ratio of EPA to DHA.

Dosage of essential fatty acids varies, but as a general rule two capsules daily is a standard dose. Omega-3 fatty acids from fish oil should be standardized to contain EPA and DHA, usually in the vicinity of 300 mg EPA and 200 mg DHA per 1,000 mg capsule of fish oil. Omega-3 fatty acids from flax oil (one tablespoon daily) are usually made from cold-pressed seed oil and contain approximately 60 percent omega-3 fatty acids.

Supplemental omega-3 oils are best tolerated when taken with food to avoid nausea and an unpleasant burping of fish oil. If you're having trouble with the odor, try freezing the capsules and taking them frozen. Individuals on blood thinning medications should alert their healthcare practitioners about their fish oil or flaxseed oil supplementation as it may affect their INR test results (tests used to adjust the medication dosage). Individuals with fish allergies should not take fish oil capsules but may benefit from plant-based omega-3 products such as algae-based oil or flaxseed oil. Plant-based supplements are also a great option for vegetarians.

PROBIOTICS

Who would think that bacteria would be one of our foundational cancer prevention recommendations? Beneficial bacteria, also known as commensal bacteria or probiotics, are in fact essential ingredients in our Five to Thrive supplement program. As we discussed in Chapter 2, we rely on these beneficial bacteria for a variety of essential functions. The bacteria in our intestinal tract help us to metabolize vitamins into their absorbable and bioactive components, bind waste products for removal in our stool, and help regulate our immunity.

Our bodies are colonized with bacteria during birth and with early breastfeeding. Afterward, we maintain bacteria through the foods we eat—particularly fermented foods such as miso, yogurt, fresh sauerkraut, and kefir. Since our bodies cannot produce bacteria, we rely upon external sources (food and supplements) to replenish and maintain the bacteria that we have. Unfortunately daily living can take its toll on the quantity and type of bacteria in our bodies.

One of the ways we destroy our beneficial bacterial population is through the use of antibiotics. While antibiotics can be immensely helpful and even life-saving, they are indiscriminate and kill many of our helpful bacteria while they're killing the bad bacteria. Unless we replace these beneficial bacteria during and after taking antibiotics, the digestive tract becomes imbalanced and overridden with harmful bacteria, creating a condition called dysbiosis. People with dysbiotic bowel lack beneficial bacteria and tend to have an overgrowth of disease-causing bacteria. Dysbiosis also leads to leaky gut, which we defined in Chapter 2. Unfortunately, as we age, our intestinal resilience decreases, and we are more susceptible to dysbiosis, intestinal inflammation, and leaky gut.

The connection between dysbiosis and our overall health is significant and far-reaching. From a cancer prevention perspective, dysbiosis significantly impacts each of the five pathways. The connection to the digestion pathway is pretty obvious. In addition to causing leaky gut syndrome, dysbiosis is strongly associated with irritable bowel syndrome. Dysbiosis also leaves our digestive tract relatively undefended against disease-causing microbes such as *Helicobacter pylori*, a causative agent of gastric ulcers.

The relationship between probiotics and our hormonal system is best illustrated in our moods. The health of our digestive tract has a surprisingly strong impact on mood—especially depression and anxiety. We have long known that stress, depression, and anxiety can aggravate intestinal disorders such as irritable bowel syndrome and inflammatory bowel disease. One mechanism for this is that stress can cause reductions in *Lactobacillus* and *Bifidobacteria* species—two of the most important beneficial bacterial species in our gut. The reverse is also true, in that having enough beneficial bacteria is linked to a "good" mood. *The British Journal of Nutrition* published a fascinating double-blinded, randomized controlled trial of 55 healthy people who received either 30 days of a probiotic supplement (*Lactobacillus helveticus* and *Bifidobacterium longum*) or placebo (inactive substance). Those taking the probiotic had reduced depression, irritability, and anxiety and increased coping ability in response to stress. The probiotics reduced inflammatory chemicals (cytokines) in the gut, preventing their otherwise negative impact on neurons and mood. By altering these cytokines, probiotics improved both gut health and mood. A more stable mood results in better protection against stress-induced hormones, preserving the delicate hormonal balance essential to our health.

Probiotics also enhance our immune response. A 2009 article in *Vaccine* reviewed two trials of elderly individuals and found that flu-vaccinated individuals who also took a supplemental probiotic drink twice a day for 13 weeks demonstrated significantly increased post-vaccination antibody titers (the protective effect of the flu vaccine) compared to individuals who did not drink the probiotic. In another 2005 study in the *Journal of Clinical Nutrition*, adults who received oral probiotics had significantly decreased cold symptoms, as well as shorter duration of common cold episodes. These and other studies demonstrate the cooperative role that probiotics play in maintaining our immune defenses.

Probiotics also influence the balance of pro- and anti-inflammatory cytokines and decrease inflammatory cytokines. By doing this, probiotics exert epigenetic influences on our genome and create a less inflamed environment. Probiotics reduce oxidative stress throughout the body, which further limits inflammation and cellular damage and ultimately helps prevent cancer.

Probiotics, particularly *Bifidobacterium spp.*, also improve glucose tolerance, lower insulin levels, and maintain insulin sensitivity. Probiotics preserve intestinal integrity and maintain a healthy intestinal barrier. It is believed that this lowers inflammation and oxidative stress. The insulin receptor is very susceptible to oxidative stress; in fact, this is thought to be one of the main mechanisms underlying insulin resistance. By reducing gut-derived inflammation, probiotics lower oxidative insult to insulin receptors.

Given its direct support of each of the key pathways, probiotic use has been linked directly to cancer prevention. One clinical trial randomized 398 Japanese adults with a previous history of colon cancer to receive either dietary fiber from wheat bran or *Lactobacillus casei*, a probiotic. After four years, they were examined by colonoscopy for new tumors. Among the subjects taking the wheat bran, the risk of developing new tumors was unaffected. However, in the subjects taking lactobacillus, the chance of developing a colon cancer recurrence was reduced by 24 percent. Although the trial was small, similar results have been demonstrated in several other clinical trials. Other research suggests a protective role of probiotics on the stomach, potentially lowering the risk of stomach cancer. Some preclinical research studies suggest probiotics might reduce the risk of liver and bladder cancer.

Probiotics can be taken as single strains of *Lactobacillus* or *Bifidobacterium* or as combinations of several different bacterial species.

All of these supplements have the potential to be beneficial. The single-species probiotics work because *Lactobacillus spp.* and *Bifidobacterium spp.* are the most common and dominant bacteria in our intestines. These bacteria survive well in our intestines and when present in sufficient quantities, they create an intestinal pH that facilitates colonization by other beneficial bacteria. Combination probiotics supply a variety of the beneficial bacteria, which may facilitate the reestablishment of a healthy balance of bacteria in the bowel more quickly. Some probiotic supplements also contain prebiotics, compounds that feed and protect the beneficial bacteria. These can include things like lactoferrin, fructooligosaccharide (FOS), and a beneficial yeast known as *Saccharomyces boulardii.*

The most common quality issue related to probiotics is inadequate potency. Probiotics are living organisms, which means they eventually die. High-quality probiotic products have mechanisms in place to reduce the die off of these bacteria. Additionally to extend shelf life and viability, high-quality probiotics are packaged in blister packs or dark glass bottles. Other quality issues include inappropriate identification of the bacterial species or strain and use of a strain that has not been shown to be effective in humans. When purchasing a probiotic, it is important to make sure there is research documenting the strain's use in humans. One of the most well-respected strain of *lactobacillus acidophilus*, for instance, is a strain called NCFM. Consulting with a qualified integrative healthcare practitioner or pharmacist will provide you with guidance to obtain the best product.

We recommend Dr. Ohhira's Probiotics®, Kyo-Dophilus®, or products that contain the NCFM strain. One capsule of the Kyo-Dophilus brand has 1.5 billion colony forming units (CFUs) of the three most common bacteria. Kyo-Dophilus is unique because it is formulated with aged garlic extract, which works synergistically with probiotics. There is no recommended daily allowance for probiotics, and dosing can vary significantly depending upon the user's age, medical conditions, and medications, as well as quality of the product. Generally speaking, probiotic supplementation is recommended between 10 million and 10 billion CFU daily.

To prevent dysbiosis from antibiotic use, we recommend probiotics be taken concurrently with antibiotics and for several weeks afterwards. But then again, if you are following this plan, you are already taking probiotics on a daily basis and will continue to do so even if you are prescribed an antibiotic. It is best to take the probiotic at a different time of day than the antibiotic. Probiotics are very safe except in people who have a decreased white blood cell count (below normal). In this instance, probiotics should not be taken because of the reported risk of septicemia (blood infection).

POLYPHENOLS

As we discussed in Chapter 5, polyphenols (also called flavonoids) are one of the main reasons we advocate a colorful diet full of vegetables and fruits. Thousands of colorful flavonoids are present in foods; however, there are a few that stand out for their cancer-prevention actions. From a dietary supplement standpoint, there are three heavy hitters in the flavonoid world to be aware of:

1. Green tea flavonoid catechins and L-theanine
2. Curcumin from turmeric root
3. Resveratrol from red grape skins, peanuts, and small berries

Let's take a closer look at the unique cancer prevention profile of these flavonoids.

GREEN TEA—EGCG AND L-THEANINE

Green tea is processed from the leaves of the tea plant, *Camellia sinensis*. While all forms of traditional tea come from this plant, green tea is processed differently from black and oolong teas. For green tea, immediately after the tea leaves are picked, they are steamed to stop the fermentation process and then dried. Black tea is fermented fully by drying the leaves for many hours, rolling them to release additional enzymes, and drying further. Oolong tea is a partially fermented tea. By minimizing the fermentation process in green tea, more of the naturally present compounds found in tea are preserved. Green tea is rich in catechins (polyphenols), vitamins, minerals, and amino acids (such as L-theanine). It also has caffeine, but only about two-thirds the amount found in coffee. Caffeine content increases with additional fermentation, so black tea has more caffeine than green tea.

Of the catechins in green tea, epigallocatechin gallate, or EGCG, is the most well-studied flavonoid. Another important constituent in green tea is L-theanine, an amino acid. Green tea has been studied in humans for prevention of heart disease, obesity, and cancer. The potential benefit in these conditions is the result of green tea's effect on each of the five key pathways. Remember, this is how we prioritize the herbs and nutrients that make it to the foundation plan—how many of the pathways do they positively influence. Green tea touches all five!

The evidence supporting green tea's cancer prevention effects comes from large and small population studies. While these types of studies are not as definitive as double-blinded clinical trials, they are very helpful in assessing the long-term impact of green tea as a part of day-to-day life—which is exactly how prevention works. A good portion of the research on green tea has been done on drinking green tea as opposed to taking green tea supplements. Keep in mind that when research mentions one cup, it means a traditional Japanese cup—about 100 mL or 3.5 oz. A typical American mug of tea is about 8 oz.

Prostate cancer is perfectly suited to the prevention benefits of green tea because it typically takes decades to grow, giving ample opportunity to use targeted cancer prevention strategies like green tea over a long period of time. In a 2006 study in *Cancer Research*, 60 volunteers with high-grade prostate intraepithelial neoplasia, a precancerous condition, participated in a double-blind, placebo-controlled study. The treatment group took green tea capsules totaling 600 mg every day. After one year, only one tumor was diagnosed among the 30 men taking the green tea, whereas nine cancers were found among the 30 placebo-treated men. Total prostate-specific antigen (PSA) was lower in the green tea drinkers than in the placebo-treated men. Assuming this effect continues year after year, this indicates strong cancer prevention potential for green tea.

Cancers of the digestive tract also seem to respond to the preventive effects of green tea. In a study that looked at the health histories of 2,658 non-smoking and non-drinking adults, half of whom eventually developed esophageal cancer, those who drank green tea had almost 50 percent less likelihood of developing esophageal cancer than did those who didn't drink green tea. A similar relationship between green tea drinking and stomach cancer exists, with regular long-term green tea drinkers enjoying a 50 percent reduced risk of developing stomach cancer. A study published in the *International Journal of Cancer* found that green tea drinking reduced the incidence of chronic gastritis, or inflammation and ulceration of the stomach, which is a risk factor for stomach cancer.

A double-blind, randomized trial in a 2008 issue of *Cancer Epidemiology, Biomarkers and Prevention*, studied 136 adults with a history of colon polyps (a cancer risk factor) and assessed the impact of green tea on the development of colon cancer. The treatment group took 1,500 mg of green tea extract tablets that were standardized to 80 percent catechins and also drank six (3.5 oz) cups of green tea daily for one year. The control group only drank the green tea. After a year, all participants underwent colonoscopy. Thirty-one percent of those who did not take the tablets developed at least one colon polyp, whereas only 15 percent of the treatment group developed one or more polyp. The addition of the green tea supplement lowered the risk of colon polyps by 50 percent. This is an important study because it shows that quantity matters. By adding the capsules, the daily consumption of green tea was raised to more than 10 cups daily, a quantity that is most consistently associated with cancer prevention across all cancer types. This study also indicates the role supplements can play in boosting the level of green tea—great news for people who can't drink 10 cups of green tea every day. Plus, green tea capsules are over 99 percent caffeine-free.

Breast cancer has also been shown in population studies to respond positively to green tea. A 2001 issue of *Cancer Letters* featuring 1,160 post-surgical women with breast cancer demonstrated that those who drank three or more cups of green tea daily (average consumption was five cups daily) had a 31 percent decreased risk of breast cancer recurrence over their non-tea drinking counterparts. The protective effects from green tea regarding recurrence in the women with early (stages I and II) breast cancer equaled a 51 percent reduction. A similar effect was found in in a 1998 study in the *Japanese Journal of Cancer Research*, which studied 472 Japanese women diagnosed with breast cancer. Women who had early stage breast cancer who drank at least five cups of green tea (average of seven cups) daily had an 8 percent reduction in recurrence rate, and the recurrences were delayed by almost a full year compared to women who drank less than four cups of green tea daily (average was two cups).

A 2010 study published in *Breast Cancer Research* journal questions the breast cancer preventive actions of green tea. This study was a large study featuring more than 53,000 Japanese women living in Japan. The study followed these women for an average of 13.6 years. The participants' green tea drinking was reported in a questionnaire at the beginning of the study and then every five years. The researchers concluded that the amount of green tea consumed had no impact on the risk of breast cancer.

While the results of this study are at odds with previous research, there may be some explanations. The women in this study had a very low incidence of breast cancer, and it may be that in a population of women already at relatively low risk, frequent green tea consumption is not an impactful prevention strategy. This would mean that women at higher risk of breast cancer (like the women with a previous diagnosis of breast cancer in the earlier studies) are the ones most likely to benefit from its preventive actions. The lack of benefit in this study may also be because the typical Japanese diet is already very high in a variety of flavonoids from soy and vegetables. Adding more flavonoids such as those found in green tea may not add more benefit to a diet already rich in protection. If this is true, women eating six to eight servings of vegetables and fruits daily may not get the protective benefits from green tea, but women eating fewer servings may benefit greatly from it.

Several large population studies have demonstrated protective benefits against the development of cancers of the cervix, lung, bladder, and head and neck. Green tea supports detoxification, provides antioxidant protection, and helps create a state of relaxed alertness.

A variety of green tea supplements are available. We recommend the ingredient Sunphenon® because it is properly standardized and is made up of highly purified polyphenols found naturally in green tea. A 300 mg capsule of green tea extract that is standardized to contain at least 50 percent catechins, preferably 80 percent catechins, of which at least 45 percent is EGCG, is equivalent to two Japanese cups of tea. The Sunphenon ingredient contains greater than 80 percent polyphenols and catechins. To achieve the equivalent of 10 cups daily (assuming that you are not also drinking green tea), you would need to take four to five capsules daily. For anti-anxiety, blood pressure–lowering, and additional antioxidant effects, look for an extract standardized to contain L-theanine (Suntheanine®) at 100 mg per capsule. The typical dose of L-theanine is 200 to 300 mg. Green tea extracts should be chosen with care. Commercially grown green tea will contain pesticide residue, which can remain in the green tea extract. Green tea extract may also contain carcinogenic solvent residues. It is important to learn from the manufacturer how they ensure that each batch of their green tea extracts are solvent- and pesticide-free. Generally, the best quality green tea will be made from organically grown plants, and each batch will be screened for solvent residues.

Quality green tea extract is generally considered quite safe. However, it can alter the effectiveness of other medications such as blood thinners (Coumadin), oral contraceptives, and beta-blockers. In some people, high doses of green tea can cause anxiety, tremors, palpitations, and insomnia. Green tea can also cause weight loss, which can actually be an added benefit for some people.

CURCUMIN

Curcumin refers to a large group of flavonoids known as curcuminoids found in the root of the turmeric plant (*Curcuma longa*). Turmeric is part of the traditional diets of many Asian countries. It has

GREEN TEA AND THE FIVE PATHWAYS

Pathways	Key Findings
Immune	• **Stimulates T cells:** L-theanine is broken down to ethylamine, which specifically activates T lymphocytes to proliferate and secrete interferon gamma, increasing immune reactivity against viruses and cancer. • **Antimicrobial:** EGCG can kill bacteria and viruses, including the influenza virus.
Inflammation	• **Antioxidant:** Green tea polyphenols exert antioxidant effects, decreasing the formation of lipid peroxides (oxidants) • **Anti-inflammatory:** Epigallocatechin gallate (EGCG) inhibits the initial inflammatory response to ultraviolet-B (UVB) radiation, thereby reducing cellular damage. • **Inhibits tissue inflammation:** EGCG inhibits matrix metalloproteinases, which are released in inflamed tissue and allow inflammation to spread.
Hormones	• **Reduces the stress response:** L-theanine increases dopamine and serotonin production and generates alpha waves in the central nervous system, resulting in lower blood pressure and reduced anxiety (causing a relaxed yet alert state). • **Modulates hormonal activity in fat cells:** Inhibits fat cell proliferation and differentiation and may decrease release of obesity-related hormones.
Insulin Resistance	• **Stimulates fat oxidation:** EGCG stimulates fat metabolism into energy and has been shown in some clinical trials to support healthy weight. • **Inhibits IGF-1:** EGCG has been shown to inhibit insulin growth factor-1 activation.
Digestion and Detoxification	• **Decreases activation of carcinogens:** *In vitro* studies show that EGCG stimulates cytochrome P450 detoxification enzymes and blocks the mutagenic (DNA-damaging) effects of carcinogens.

been used in Asian and Ayurvedic systems of medicine for centuries as an anti-inflammatory, digestive aid, and liver tonic. Curcumin has been researched extensively around the world. One of the challenges with curcumin is that it is poorly absorbed from the digestive tract into the blood. As little as 15 percent (perhaps up to 60 percent) of orally consumed curcumin is absorbed intact. Due to the poor absorption profile of curcumin, very few clinical studies have been conducted to determine if the wide range of activities of curcumin seen in pre-clinical studies are applicable in humans. This is changing now with the development of specialized preparations of termeric that enhance the absorption and bioavailability of curcumin.

In vitro (test tube) and animal studies have shown that curcumin inhibits cancer formation at all stages of development; it protects cells against initial damage from cancer-causing compounds, slows tumor growth, stimulates apoptosis of cancer cells, and prevents the formation of blood vessels necessary for tumor growth. Curcumin has been shown to inhibit the growth of colon, breast, prostate, and melanoma cancer cell lines.

Curcumin has also been studied clinically in humans. Curcumin extract has been shown in clinical trials to inhibit the growth of colon and pancreatic cancers. The trials are small and preliminary, and the impact of curcumin from a prevention standpoint is not well understood. However, given the pronounced anticancer effect of curcumin seen in in vitro and animal studies and the vast number of genes and pathways that curcumin modifies, the prevention potential for curcumin is significant. A 2006 study in *Clinical Gastroenterology and Hepatology* demonstrating this potential was done on people with familial adenomatous polyposis (FAP), which is a risk factor for colon cancer. In this study, five patients with FAP received 480 mg of curcumin and 20 mg of quercetin (another plant-derived flavonoid) orally three times daily for six months before colon removal. The number of polyps decreased by 60 percent and the size of polyps decreased by 50 percent in the removed colons. These patients tolerated the treatment well and without side effects. Another human study published in *Anticancer Research* in 2001 found that of 25 individuals

CURCUMIN AND THE FIVE PATHWAYS

Pathways	Key Findings
Immune	• **Reduces T-cell–induced inflammation:** Curcumin inhibits T-cell NF-kB activation (animal study) • **Antimicrobial:** Turmeric extract and the essential oil of Curcuma longa inhibit the growth of a variety of bacteria, parasites, and pathogenic fungi.
Inflammation	• **Antioxidant:** *In vitro* studies have shown that curcuminoids exert potent antioxidant effects and enhance cellular resistance to oxidative damage. • **Anti-inflammatory:** Curcuminoids exert liver-protective effects, in part due to reduced production of inflammatory cytokines. • **Inhibits NF-kB:** Curcumin potently down-regulates NF-kB and in so doing inhibits the amplification of the inflammatory response.
Hormones	• **Increases resistance to stress:** Curcumin is effective in alleviating chronic stress-induced disorders in rodents by modulating neuroendocrine functions of the central nervous system. • **Modifies cortisol secretion:** Curcumin inhibits cortisol secretion stimulated by ACTH, which helps reestablish the sensitivity of the stress response axis.
Insulin Resistance	• **Reduces insulin resistance:** *In vitro* and animal studies have shown that curcumin down-regulates the inflammatory cytokines resistin and leptin and up-regulates adiponectin, as well as altering signal transduction pathways. The net effect of these actions is a reversal of insulin resistance, high blood sugar, elevated lipids, and other inflammatory symptoms associated with obesity and metabolic diseases.
Digestion and Detoxification	• **Improves digestion:** Curcumin inhibits intestinal spasm and increases digestive enzyme secretion (animal studies). • **Protects against ulcer formation:** Turmeric has been shown in animals to inhibit ulcer formation caused by stress, alcohol, and medications. This effect has been demonstrated in a clinical trial of 25 patients with endoscopically diagnosed gastric ulcer. Six hundred milligrams of powdered turmeric five times daily resulted in complete healing of the ulcers after 12 weeks of treatment. • **Supports detoxification:** Curcumin exerts potent antioxidant effects in the liver, protecting liver cells from oxidative stress and increases bile output and solubility, which supports the elimination of fat-soluble toxins.

at high risk of cancer who had pre-malignant lesions, there was a decreased progression of cancer in 50 percent of patients with recently surgically removed bladder cancer, 28 percent of patients with oral leukoplakia (a precancerous condition of the mouth), 16 percent of patients with intestinal metaplasia of the stomach (a precancerous condition of the stomach), and 25 percent patients with cervical intraepithelial neoplasm (a precancerous condition of the cervix). Although more clinical trials are needed to further determine the direct potential of curcumin specific to cancer prevention, because it positively influences all five pathways it is a foundational supplement in our plan. "Curcumin is one of the most widely studied polyphenols, and impacts multiple pathways in various human cancers," concludes Ajay Goel, PhD, curcumin researcher and Director of Epigenetics and Cancer Prevention at Baylor University Medical Center.

One of the challenges with curcumin supplementation is finding a form that is absorbable and bioavailable. Because of this challenge we are careful to only recommend an ingredient and brand that has proven bioavailability and scientific research. BCM-95® is a proprietary micronized form of curcumin blended with turmeric essential oils. The mixture enhances absorption and delays elimination, resulting in significantly enhanced bioavailability. In a pilot crossover study, BCM-95 demonstrated six times better absorption compared to a curcumin-lecithin-piperine formula and seven to ten times better absorption than plain curcumin. Of note, curcumin supplements with piperine are not recommended since piperine interacts with a wide spectrum of prescription medications as well as increases the absorption of other toxins from the digestive tract. Any form of curcumin should be tested to be free of solvent residues, pesticides, and heavy metals. These tests should be made available to you upon request for the lot of any curcumin product that you purchase. In natural health stores, you can find BCM-95 under the name CuraMed® in the Terry Naturally brand, and through healthcare professionals CuraPro™ in the *EuroMedica* brand contains this special form of curcumin (both are distributed in North American by EuroPharma, Inc.).

The dosage of curcumin for prevention is largely unknown. The few prevention studies that have been done have demonstrated benefit with ranges of 480 mg to 2,000 mg of curcumin. Correlating these results with the absorption data of BCM-95, a daily dosage of one to two capsules of BCM-95 should result in sufficient curcumin to exert preventive effects.

Curcumin is well-tolerated, other than causing occasional mild digestive upset. Curcumin inhibits certain cytochrome P450 detoxification enzymes (CYP1A2) and enhances others (CYP2A6), so it may interfere with other medications. If you are taking medications, it is important to consult with a qualified integrative healthcare practitioner or a pharmacist before starting curcumin.

ANTIOXIDANTS

Antioxidants are the fourth part of our Five to Thrive supplement foundation program. While diet should be your major source of antioxidants, it can be difficult to obtain enough antioxidants to meet the oxidative challenge of daily living. We live in a world of oxidative stress. We are exposed to many of the more than 100,000 chemicals in regular use through the air we breathe, the water we drink, and the materials and products we come in contact with. In fact, the vast majority of us have environmental chemicals in our body tissues. These chemicals are reactive and destructive. Accumulation of these toxic compounds plays a role in the development of most chronic diseases, including cancer.

Our bodies are designed to generate antioxidants to combat the oxidants we are exposed to on a daily basis. The most important internal antioxidant, glutathione, is found in every cell in the body, in large measure to neutralize the oxidative damage of daily living. Unfortunately, with the added burden of environmental toxins, it is far too easy to overwhelm our antioxidant defenses. This can leave our cells susceptible to damage that ultimately leads to disease, cancer included.

So how do these important antioxidants work? Antioxidants bind to toxins so they can be safely eliminated. When an oxidative

WHAT ABOUT HOMEOPATHY?

Homeopathy, also known as homeopathic medicine, is a system of diagnosis and treatment based upon the principle of similars, or "like cures like." Homeopathy was developed in Germany in the 1800s and is practiced worldwide. Homeopathy is used for wellness and prevention and to treat many diseases and conditions. Our colleague Dr. Nancy Gahles, who is a gifted homeopathic practitioner and chiropractor, explains it this way: "The philosophy of homeopathic therapeutics involves all the principles of healthy living as disease prevention, including, diet, lifestyle, hygiene, environment, stress management, and positive relationships. The selection of a well-suited homeopathic remedy, according to the principles of homeopathic laws, has the potential to stimulate the organism to a gentle, rapid, permanent restoration of health."

The basic idea of homeopathy is that a disease or constitutional imbalance can be corrected by minute amounts of a substance that, if given in its full dose, would produce symptoms similar to that being expressed by the disease or imbalance. Homeopathy has been the subject of clinical research with positive findings in a number of conditions. Homeopathy is also safe and can be helpful in restoring physical, mental, and emotional well-being as a part of a comprehensive cancer prevention plan. It is important to receive homeopathic guidance and recommendations from a qualified homeopathic provider. The following certifications require training and testing in homeopathy (for more information refer to the resource section of the book):

CCH: Certified by the Council for Homeopathic Certification

RSHom (NA): Registered by the North American Society of Homeopaths

DHANP: Diplomate of the Homeopathic Academy of Naturopathic Physicians

DHt: Diplomate in Homeotherapeutics by the American Board of Homeotherapeutics.

---

reactive molecule, called a free radical, encounters an antioxidant, it is neutralized. Antioxidants also trigger defensive mechanisms inside damaged cells. If a cell has undergone extensive oxidative damage, particularly to its DNA, the cell must either repair itself or, if the damage is too great, undergo apoptosis (cell suicide). Many antioxidants stimulate cell repair and apoptosis.

Antioxidants also support and enhance the health of all five pathways, most notably inflammation. Inflammation is essentially an oxidative process that causes damage. Chronic inflammation happens when that chain of reactive free radical–induced damage continues unhindered. Antioxidants are one of the most effective ways to stop chronic inflammation, because oxidative damage and inflammation are inextricably intertwined. By reducing underlying oxidation, the antioxidants help prevent chronic diseases such as cancer.

Antioxidants are also important in maintaining immunity. They activate natural killer (NK) cells and stimulate immune cells to increase phagocytosis (the engulfing and ingestion of bacteria or other foreign bodies by immune cells). Phagocytosis requires that the immune cell produce free radicals to inject into the foreign body to destroy it. Given the danger posed to the immune cell itself, antioxidants are necessary to regulate the reactions that release free radicals. Immune cells are most active if they have sufficient stores of glutathione, the master antioxidant. Glutathione deficiency impairs T cell reactivity.

Insulin resistance is, in many respects, the result of oxidative damage as well, because the insulin receptor is vulnerable to damage from environmental toxins. This is illustrated by the fact that obese people who do have elevated environmental toxins in their bodies have increased risk of developing diabetes. Obese people with low levels of environmental toxins are not at as high of an increased risk of developing diabetes compared to those with a higher toxin burden. This means that environmental toxin load can be a stronger diabetes risk factor than obesity. This also means that antioxidants, particularly glutathione, are critical for reducing this oxidative damage, thereby reducing insulin resistance and diabetes risk.

From a hormonal standpoint, endocrine glands are quite sensitive to oxidative damage. For example, thyroid function is dependent upon the antioxidant nutrient coenzyme Q10 (CoQ10), and the hypothalamic-pituitary-adrenal axis is dependent upon overall antioxidant status. Oxidative stress has been implicated in thyroid disease, adrenal dysfunction, and reproductive issues. Environmental oxidative chemicals such as bisphenol A (BPA) also impact estrogen driven processes. BPA binds to, and stimulates, the estrogen receptor, potentially driving estrogen receptor–positive cancer growth. Antioxidant therapy helps protect against endocrine disrupters such as BPA.

Antioxidants are critical to digestive health and proper detoxification, because they help preserve the health of the intestinal mucosa, maintain sufficient secretion of digestive enzymes, and promote proper bowel function. Antioxidants also quench the oxidants that are created during the first phase of detoxification, which protects us from oxidative damage. Antioxidants are also used to bind and eliminate oxidative compounds that emerge from phase I detoxification. The antioxidants used to bind and eliminate oxidants are in constant demand, particularly in light of our ongoing exposure to environmental pollutants.

The importance of antioxidants in cancer prevention cannot be overstated. After all, antioxidants are the main mechanism of action in most of the cancer prevention research regarding diet. Not all antioxidants are created equal, and in the case of cancer prevention, the most important antioxidants are glutathione and CoQ10. Glutathione is critical for elimination of environmental pollutants, which lowers all types of cancer risk. CoQ10 is associated with decreased risk of cancers of the breast and thyroid, as well as melanoma. Vitamin C is associated with lower risk of gastric cancer. Vitamin E and selenium, although important antioxidants, have not been shown in clinical studies to decrease cancer risk. Certainly there are other antioxidants that show promise as well, however, it is our goal to help you prioritize the ones that will influence as many pathways as possible and have strong scientific substantiation.

Oral glutathione—which is available as a supplement—has been shown in clinical trials to create antioxidant effects systemically. Oral glutathione is absorbed intact, is broken down into its three amino acids (glutamic acid, cysteine, and glycine) and then reassembled in the target organs, or is used up by the intestinal cells themselves. However, not all glutathione supplements are created equal. We recommend the Setria® brand ingredient as an efficient way to replenish depleted glutathione stores. This is a high-quality and nontoxic ingredient. Look for it on the label of any product containing glutathione. A 100–200 mg dose of glutathione in the morning is optimal, since our glutathione levels are at their lowest level in the morning. It is also possible to raise intracellular glutathione by taking nutrients that the body uses to make glutathione. These nutrients include alpha lipoic acid, selenium, and n-acetyl cysteine.

CoQ10, or ubiquinone, is also available as a supplement. Some cholesterol-lowering drugs, particularly statins, have been shown to lower blood levels of CoQ10, so people taking these medications should also take CoQ10. There are no known contraindications to taking CoQ10, though it can sometimes cause mild nausea and diarrhea, especially at doses above 200 mg. CoQ10 is best absorbed when taken with a meal. Typically 30–100 mg is sufficient for prevention purposes. Unfortunately, CoQ10 products can be adulterated with a fake CoQ10 compound. Make sure the CoQ10 product you are using has been tested for adulteration. To prevent oxidation, use a branded CoQ10 such as Kaneka QH® reduced form of CoQ10 or Kyolic Formula 110 that combines aged garlic extract with 60 mg of CoQ10.

As we mentioned in the diet chapter, another powerful antioxidant is garlic. From a dietary supplement standpoint, perhaps the most widely studied garlic (from a broad perspective, including cardiovascular and immune stimulation) is aged garlic extract. So far, data directly linking ingestion of garlic and cancer prevention is somewhat limited; however, preliminary *in vitro* studies show that compounds found in garlic can induce apoptosis in certain cancer cells such as colon, prostate, and esophageal. Aged garlic extract directly influences the inflammatory, immune, and digestion/detoxification pathways. We recommend Kyolic brand aged garlic extract because it is made from 100 percent organically grown garlic bulbs that are aged using a unique extraction process that eliminates odor. Kyolic also has a unique super-fruit powder called Kyo-Red that has high polyphenol content to provide supplemental antioxidants from colorful fruits that are so important.

VITAMIN D

Let's wrap up this list with a little sunshine—the sunshine vitamin that is. Vitamin D is our fifth foundational dietary supplement because of the numerous studies highlighting its importance to our health. Vitamin D3 is a fat-soluble vitamin produced by the body. This production starts when our skin is exposed to sunlight. Vitamin D is also found in foods such as fish and fish oil (especially cod liver oil), eggs, and fortified milk.

Vitamin D is a hormonal vitamin, meaning there are receptors for vitamin D in the body. In fact, every cell has vitamin D receptors on its surface. When vitamin D binds to these receptors, various processes are initiated in our cells that translate into a variety of actions. While we don't understand the role of vitamin D in every organ, we know that it is necessary for maintaining our blood and bone levels of calcium and phosphorus. Vitamin D deficiency results in increased bone loss and increases the rate of falls and fracture, especially in the elderly. Vitamin D supports immune function, and deficiency results in more colds and flu. Vitamin D promotes cell maturation and regulates inflammation, and deficiency increases the risk of cancer and autoimmune disease. Vitamin D is used in the production of neurotransmitters in our brain and deficiency is linked to depression.

The role of vitamin D in maintaining the health of each of the five pathways can be summarized as follows.

Most of our vitamin D comes from exposure to sunlight. However, this source is compromised at northern latitudes and during the fall and winter months. Sunscreens and clothing also prevent vitamin D from entering our bodies. Skin-derived synthesis of vitamin D also varies from person to person depending upon the pigmentation of the skin, age, sunscreen use, and amount of skin exposed to the sun. Vitamin D deficiency is more common among African Americans than Caucasians, for instance, because of greater pigmentation of darker skin. Obese people also tend to be more vitamin D–deficient than non-obese individuals. Vitamin D levels are also compromised in people with inflammatory digestive diseases and in people with dysbiosis, because they are not able to efficiently absorb vitamin D from dietary sources.

Vitamin D insufficiency, which may or may not be accompanied by symptoms, is linked to several health problems, including cancer. The role of vitamin D insufficiency in cancer prevention is emerging as an important rationale for vitamin D testing and potentially supplementation.

Vitamin D has been studied in many large population studies that show people with the lowest levels of vitamin D are at increased risk for developing cancers of the colon, breast, prostate, and pancreas, as well as non-Hodgkins lymphoma. Even more alarming is the fact that many of these studies have shown that vitamin D insufficiency is linked with higher cancer fatality. A 2007 trial in the *American Journal of Clinical Nutrition* of over 1,000 healthy postmenopausal women was conducted over four years showing that women who took 1,500 mg of calcium with 1,100 IU of vitamin D had a lower incidence of all types of cancer compared to the women who took a placebo.

Another double-blind, randomized controlled trial in a 2009 issue of *Cancer Prevention Research* showed that adults who took 800 IU of vitamin D daily had more apoptotic (cell death) gene expression in the colon compared to placebo. This study determined that although vitamin D and calcium were effective at increasing apoptosis, vitamin D was the most effective. A 2007 meta-analysis of different studies in the *American Journal of Preventive Medicine* concluded that higher blood levels of vitamin D were associated with a 50 percent lower risk of colorectal cancer. The authors further conclude that daily intake of 1,000–2,000 IU/day of vitamin D3 could reduce the incidence of colorectal cancer with minimal risk.

A 2007 review of several studies on colon, ovary, and breast cancer found that maintaining blood level of vitamin D at or above 42 ng/mL would result in prevention of 30 percent of breast cancers. Women with a history of breast cancer should certainly pay attention to their vitamin D levels, as low vitamin D levels have been associated with a faster progression of metastatic breast cancer. To make this even more significant, vitamin D insufficiency is more common among women with previously diagnosed breast cancer. This same study found that nearly 38 percent of women were defi-

VITAMIN D AND THE FIVE PATHWAYS

Pathways	Key Findings
Immune	• **Suppresses auto-immunity:** Immune cells activate vitamin D and express the vitamin D receptor on their surfaces. Vitamin D affects the activity of all immune cells—T cells, B cells, and antigen-presenting cells (dendritic cells and macrophages). The overall effect of vitamin D on the immune system is to suppress auto-immune reactivity.
Inflammation	• **Anti-inflammatory:** Deficiency of vitamin D increases the risk of almost all inflammatory diseases. Vitamin D deficiency is linked with increased inflammatory cytokines, specifically CRP, IL-6, and TNF-*a*. • **Inhibits inflammatory cytokines:** Vitamin D has been shown to inhibit the influx of inflammatory cytokines in distressed tissues.
Hormones	• **Steroidal hormone:** The effects of vitamin D in the body are hormonal ones, and as with other hormones, there are receptors in cells for vitamin D. Vitamin D influences bone density via hormone-like signaling. • **Exerts antidepressant actions:** Vitamin D insufficiency is also linked with anxiety and depression.
Insulin Resistance	• **Vitamin D deficiency is linked with insulin resistance:** Low blood levels of vitamin D are associated with metabolic syndrome. Obese individuals with low vitamin D levels are at increased risk for developing insulin resistance.
Digestion and Detoxification	• **Gut homeostasis:** Vitamin D plays an important role in gut homeostasis and in signaling between the bacteria in our digestive tract and our tissues. • **Maintains healthy gut bacteria:** Vitamin D is essential to maintaining healthy bacteria in the digestive tract.

cient and nearly 39 percent were insufficient, which means that a combined 76 percent, or two-thirds of all women with a history of breast cancer may require increased vitamin D.

Prostate cancer has also been linked to vitamin D insufficiency. A 2007 study in *Cancer Epidemiology, Biomarkers and Prevention* found that frequent recreational sun exposure in adulthood was associated with a 53 percent reduced risk of fatal prostate cancer. Several other studies have confirmed that low blood levels of vitamin D are linked with increased incidence of prostate cancer and increased progression. In a 13-year-long study of more than 19,000 men in Finland, low vitamin D (less than 16 ng/mL) was associated with 70 percent increased rate of prostate cancer.

There is considerable debate among practitioners and researchers about the proper and optimal vitamin D dosage. Some have suggested that amounts as high as 10,000 IU each day are safe and necessary. This dose is based on the fact that whole-body sunlight exposure can result in at least 10,000 IU per day of vitamin D. However, such a high dose has not been demonstrated to be safe. When our skin is exposed to sunlight, many different vitamin D metabolites are created that regulate each other. When we take such a high dose, this regulation is not available, so oral intake is very different than high intake from the sun.

For decades, it was assumed that 400 IU of vitamin D was sufficient. Today, that is considered too low for the majority of adults. Researchers, healthcare practitioners, and large institutional organizations agree that most adults who have insufficient vitamin D levels will require at least 800 IU daily. Most researchers and practitioners have targeted 1,200 IU to 2,000 IU daily as an optimal dosage range needed to increase vitamin D into the normal range. Long-term dosage of 2,000 IU daily has also been shown in a variety of studies to be safe and well-tolerated. Doses higher than this should only be consumed under the guidance of a doctor. Your doctor will measure your blood level of vitamin D to help determine your optimal dosage and will use your vitamin D test along with other parameters of your health to determine if your dosage is appropriate. Doctors can also guide you to reliable vitamin D products. Vitamin D should be used with caution in patients taking digoxin, because hypercalcemia (which may result with excess vitamin D use) may cause abnormal heart rhythms.

Keep in mind, getting some time in the sun (but not in excess) is an excellent way to increase vitamin D levels. If you expose your arms and legs or your hands, arms, and face to sunlight for five to 15 minutes two to three times each week between 10:00 a.m. and 3:00 p.m. during the spring, summer, and autumn months, you should have sufficient vitamin D levels without getting sunburned. If you are in the sun for more than 15 minutes, wear sunscreen. Of course, if you are very fair-skinned or have a history of skin cancer, limit your sun exposure completely. That said, for the majority of us, some sun is not dangerous and is in fact good for us.

THE IMPORTANCE OF INDIVIDUALIZATION

We've used the five pathways and the concept of epigenetics to help you prioritize your supplement choices. But in the end, gaining as much information as you can and individualizing your approach is the best option of all. And you don't have to do that alone. Naturopathic doctors, holistic medical doctors, integrative nurse practitioners, chiropractors, holistic dieticians, nutritionists, and many pharmacists can help you. There are many qualified providers with training in dietary supplements who can guide you to making the most effective, safe, and individualized choices.

Remember the Five to Thrive dietary supplement ingredients featured provide a great foundation, but don't limit yourself to just those. Following is a short list of supplements that can provide additional support to each of the pathways:

- *Immunity:* mushrooms (e.g., maitake, shiitake, Ganoderma, agaricus), yeast-derived beta-glucan, zinc, echinacea

- *Inflammation:* Boswellia, tocotrienols, holy basil, ginger, resveratrol

- **Hormonal Health:** genistein, phosphatidylserine, homeopathics, 5-hydroxy tryptophan, black cohosh
- **Insulin Resistance:** magnesium, B vitamins, chromium, *Gymnema sylvestre*
- **Digestion & Detoxification:** herbal bitters, digestive enzymes, milk thistle, glycine

Dietary supplements are an important tool of modern healthcare and are a critical component of the Five to Thrive plan.

HIGH FIVE TIP *Three-legged stools are known to be one of the most solid pieces of furniture built. Using this metaphor, think of one leg of your cancer prevention plan as your diet, the second as your lifestyle and activity levels, and the third leg as your psychological and spiritual wellbeing. These three legs create a sturdy health foundation. Only when this foundation is built do you have someplace to set your supplements on!*

DISCLOSURE STATEMENT

As you will notice, we have mentioned a few specific dietary supplement brands. It is important to note that we are not paid spokespeople for any of the brands mentioned in this book, and we do not receive payment associated with any product sales. We recommend branded ingredients or specific products when we are aware of compelling advantages, significant research, or superior quality. We recommend ingredients and brands we trust. However, two of the ingredient suppliers we recommend in the book do support our Thrivers educational initiative (www.five2thrive.com) and those are Kyowa Hakko (Setria®) and Taiyo International (Suntheanine® and Sunphenon®).

CHAPTER

SCREENING STRATEGIES AND TUNE UPS

ometimes it's easier to take care of our car, home, family, and pets than it is to take care of ourselves. Every 3,000 miles we get the oil changed in the car, each winter we have the furnace looked at, we take the dog to the vet once a year, we get the kids ready for school in the fall, and we remind loved ones about important health appointments. But when it comes to our own "tune-up," there is a tendency to put it on the back burner.

We consistently hear two different trains of thought when it comes to going to the doctor, and they sound like this:

1. "I'm too busy. There's nothing wrong with me. I'll go next year."

2. "I'm afraid. What if they find something?"

The first response, while perhaps true, is also an expression of denial that is really another version of the second response. The fear expressed in the second response often comes from those who've had a previous diagnosis of cancer. We know how that feels—that sinking and shocking feeling when you hear those words "You have cancer." It's our mission to keep those words as far away from you as possible. The integrative cancer prevention plan we've described will help give you the confidence you need to work proactively with your team of healthcare professionals. You can transform your relationship with your doctors and the doctor visit by taking charge of your health (for more information, refer to the sidebar on page 178). The Five to Thrive plan will also give you the strength and resolve to tackle whatever is discovered along your journey.

Also remember the way you handle your health has far-reaching effects. How you carry out your cancer prevention plan will set the tone for your entire family and your network of friends. You can lead by example, allowing your actions to loudly send the right message to those you influence.

Whether or not you've had a previous diagnosis, this chapter will help you create a practical, effective plan that includes proper screening and integrative healthcare. We will begin by addressing basic screening. Screening tests are designed to look for cancer before symptoms arise. The goal of screening is to rule out cancer or catch it early. Please keep in mind that if your doctor recommends a screening test, it doesn't mean that you have cancer. If your screening test is abnormal, you may have to have additional tests. These are called diagnostic tests.

Before we take a closer look at screening, let's review some of the symptoms that should send you to the telephone to book an appointment with your doctor.

While these symptoms do not necessarily mean that you have cancer, they can be signs of cancer. Cancer is always most curable when it is diagnosed early, so it is a good idea to take these symptoms seriously.

- Unexplained, persistent, and worsening pain
- Extreme tiredness
- Unexplained weight loss (this includes desirable weight loss, but still unrelated to specific diet or exercise changes)
- Night sweats and fever
- Unexplained changes in your bowel frequency, or blood in your stool or urine
- A worsening dry cough (not associated with a cold or bronchitis)
- Unexplained and long-lasting voice hoarseness
- Skin pigmentation changes, yellowness, a bleeding mole, or itchiness

Should you develop any of these symptoms, see your doctor for a diagnostic work-up. In addition to following up on specific symptoms, it is important to activate a regular screening program. Let's look at screening, beginning with the colon and working our way north.

COLON

It is estimated that 90 percent of individuals diagnosed with colon cancer are over age 50. That's why both men and women should have a colonoscopy at age 50. With this test, the doctor uses a flexible tube with a miniature camera on the end to look inside the colon and rectum. This test is designed to find benign polyps, a risk factor for cancer, as well as cancerous tumors. A yearly fecal occult blood test should also be performed beginning at age 50. The fecal occult blood test is a noninvasive test that, if done every two years, will find enough cancers at an early stage to reduce death rates from colon cancer by 16 percent. This is a home-test that your doctor will provide to you. Two samples are collected from one to three consecutive stools, depending upon the type of stool test. The samples are applied to a specially prepared card. These cards are then analyzed by a laboratory for microscopic signs of blood, which can indicate the presence of cancer, inflammation, or ulceration of the digestive tract.

While colon cancer is the second most deadly cancer, it is also highly treatable when caught early. Colon cancer screening is critical and reduces death from colon cancer by up to 80 percent. After your initial colonoscopy, you should have some type of testing every five years that can include:

- Flexible sigmoidoscopy
- Double-contrast barium enema
- CT colonography (virtual colonoscopy)

If any of the above tests are positive, a colonoscopy should be performed.

If you have a family history of colon cancer or have symptoms that indicate there may be a problem, you should talk to your doctor about doing a colonoscopy before age 50.

PROSTATE

Prostate-specific antigen (PSA) is a protein that is produced in the prostate to help liquefy semen. Some of those proteins make

TRANSFORMING THE DOCTOR VISIT

By Karolyn

My sister had been cancer-free for well over a decade, so when I got her call I was shocked beyond words. I stopped breathing as she told me they found a lump, went in for a biopsy, and that she had cancer again. She was instantly hurled back in time, reliving her first diagnosis while grappling with the horror of another.

She was crying, and the only thing I could focus on was trying to find a way to be with her. We didn't live near each other. I was obsessed with rearranging my schedule and finding a way to get to her quickly.

When we were together, strategizing, talking, and even laughing until we cried, the world seemed right again. We could do this. So we started checking things off the list. She needed to find an oncologist, so she began the *interview process*. Yes, I said *interview process*. My sister wanted to work with someone who would be open to an integrative treatment. She wanted to create a partnership with her doctors and in this way, she took an important step in transforming her healthcare experience. Very few people enjoy going to doctor's appointments, whether it is for a checkup or for a follow-up, and this is even truer when a serious illness like cancer is involved.

I was with her as she interviewed her first potential doctor. "I'd like to use an integrative approach that includes dietary changes, exercise, and dietary supplements," my sister explained. Her doctor replied, "There is no evidence that any of that will help you. Your only option is chemotherapy, and you really should start quickly." With indescribable courage, confidence, and grace my sister stood up, thanked the doctor, and said, "We'll let you know." In the parking lot, she looked at me, smiled, and said, "I'm so glad I'll never see that doctor again."

On the next interview, my sister took a copy our first book, *The Definitive Guide to Cancer* and gave it to the doctor and said, "This is the approach I want to use: chemotherapy, but also support with diet, lifestyle, and dietary supplements." The doctor admitted she didn't know a lot about this approach but said "we will work together." That's the doctor my sister chose. She also worked very closely with Dr. Alschuler. Following her surgery, she also saw an acupuncturist and a physical therapist. She created a team of healthcare professionals working together on her behalf, but she was in charge. My sister transformed her healthcare experience even under very difficult circumstances. We can all follow her example—I know I do!

their way into the bloodstream. Cancerous prostate tissue cells make more PSA than benign cells; however, benign prostate cells also produce PSA. While it's true that elevated PSA levels can indicate cancer, they can also be elevated in men who have prostatitis (inflamed prostate) or an enlarged prostate (benign prostatic hyperplasia—BPH). Conversely, PSA levels may be in the normal range even when cancer is present. So you can already see the dilemma that can be created with this screening test.

Testing for elevated PSA in the blood is the only prostate cancer–screening test presently available, but because PSA can be elevated for other reasons, recommendations regarding PSA screening vary. At a minimum, most experts agree that the PSA test should not be the sole screening method. An elevated PSA should not be used as the only factor in determining if cancer is present. A high PSA number should also not be used as the only reason to do biopsies or use aggressive anticancer treatments.

Two key studies released in 2011 in prestigious journals (the *British Medical Journal* and the *Journal of Clinical Oncology*) both describe the dangers of excessive PSA screening. The study featured in the *British Medical Journal* demonstrated that screening does not reduce the risk of dying from prostate cancer; the researchers go so far as to say, "There is no escaping the fact that we need a better tool…to help detect prostate cancers that actually need treating, as opposed to innocent ones that do not." Many prostate cancers are slow moving and not life-threatening and do not warrant harsh treatments with serious side effects. PSA screening is an issue that needs to be discussed in detail with your doctor.

In addition to a digital rectal exam performed by a physician, these other factors should be considered along with the PSA level:

- Size of the prostate gland
- Speed at which PSA levels are changing
- Medications that may affect PSA, such as finasteride (Proscar), dutasteride (Avodart), and even some herbal extracts such as saw palmetto
- Age

The age at which a PSA screening test should be done has been hotly debated. As we've explained, the PSA is not a definitive test and is not necessarily associated with a reduced risk of dying from prostate cancer. Additionally, many prostate cancers are contained to the prostate are slow-growing and do not require treatment. If a slow-growing cancer is detected by an elevated PSA, this man is faced with anxiety-provoking decisions regarding a cancer that may not even be life-threatening. Prostate cancer treatment may come with serious side effects, including incontinence, erectile dysfunction, and bowel disorders. For these reasons, the PSA screening test is not generally recommended for men under the age of 50. For men who are African American, have a family history of prostate cancer in any their first-degree relatives, or who have had some prostate health issues, a PSA test before age 50 may be recommended. PSA testing is not likely necessary for men over age 75.

This can be a confusing issue, especially since the PSA test is the only screening test available. According to the American Cancer Society, "Asymptomatic men who have at least a 10-year life expectancy have an opportunity to make an informed decision with their healthcare provider about screening for prostate cancer after they receive information about the uncertainties, risks, and potential benefits associated with prostate cancer screening." In other words, talk this over with your doctor and be sure to explore all of the pros and cons of screening. Here is our bottom line: Men who are not at high risk for prostate cancer—meaning they are not African American, do not have a family history of prostate cancer in their fathers or brothers before the age of 50, and are not experiencing symptoms of prostate disorders—then it is best to avoid the PSA test until the age of 50, and even then it may not be indicated.

The testing schedule depends on initial PSA values:

- Yearly PSA screening for men whose PSA level is 2.5 ng/mL to 4.0 ng/mL, or individualized depending on other health factors.

- PSA screening every two years for men whose PSA is less than 2.5 ng/mL.

PSA greater than 4.0 ng/mL requires additional diagnostic evaluation, which may include biopsy.

PSA screening is a great illustration of the frustrating gray areas associated with cancer prevention and treatment. When it comes to issues of screening and cancer treatment, there are no easy answers, and decisions are not as clear-cut as we would like them to be. In these cases, getting as much information as possible and then applying that information to your individual circumstance is critical.

OVARIAN

While cancer screening holds great promise for many cancers, the options for ovarian cancers are extremely limited, and unfortunately these are difficult cancers to detect and treat. There is no standard screening test presently available for ovarian cancer. Some people confuse the tumor market test that evaluates circulating levels of CA-125 (a protein shed into the blood from ovarian cancer cells, but also from inflamed tissues) with screening; however, this is not a routine screening test. An increased level of CA-125 in the blood can indicate cancer; however, other noncancerous conditions such as uterine fibroids, endometriosis, and even pregnancy can increase CA-125 levels. What's more, CA-125 levels may not be increased with early-stage ovarian cancers, so they can give a false sense of security. The CA-125 test is most effectively used as a part of a diagnostic work-up and after diagnosis of ovarian cancer to track treatment success or progression of the disease.

The best way to "screen" for ovarian cancer is by understanding your risk factors and getting an annual gynecological exam. Here are some factors that can increase your risk of developing ovarian cancer:

- Family history, especially in a mother or sister
- Testing positive for the BRCA genes
- Use of hormone replacement therapy or fertility drugs
- Obesity

In addition to risk factors, it's important to know some symptoms that could be caused by ovarian cancer, but keep in mind that these symptoms do not necessarily mean you have ovarian cancer. The following symptoms, if unexplained, should be discussed with your doctor:

- Abdominal pressure or bloating
- Changes in bowel or bladder habits
- Abdominal weight gain with clothes fitting more tightly around your waist
- Low-back pain
- Persistent indigestion, gas, or nausea
- Changes in menstruation, such as irregular or heavy bleeding

In the case of suspicious symptoms, your doctor may recommend a transvaginal ultrasound and CA-125 test. Ovarian tumors, as well as benign ovarian cysts, are best detected with transvaginal ultrasound. If you have high risk factors, such as testing positive for the BRCA gene mutations, you may want to discuss getting a transvaginal ultrasound done in conjunction with a CA-125 test and your annual physical.

Ovarian cancer is the fifth most deadly cancer affecting women. Being proactive about risk factors and symptoms is absolutely critical when it comes to preventing ovarian cancer.

CERVIX AND UTERUS

The cervix connects the uterus to the vagina and is sometimes referred to as the neck of the uterus. Cervical cancer screening is done during an annual gynecological exam. Annual gynecological exams, also referred to as pelvic exams, begin within a couple of years after active vaginal intercourse but no later than age 21. During the pelvic exam, your healthcare practitioner will conduct a Pap test. This involves swabbing the cervix to collect cells for laboratory testing for precancerous changes or cancer. Also during the pelvic exam, your practitioner will conduct a bimanual exam to check other female organs such as the ovaries and uterus. A rectal exam may also be done after the bimanual exam. And, a urine test

REDUCING RADIATION WORRIES

Some screening tests, like CT scans, mammograms, MRIs, and X-rays, increase our exposure to radiation, which could theoretically increase our risk of developing cancer. And yet, these are valid tests that are often necessary to help rule out cancer or catch it early. Some health-care practitioners may tell you the exposure is minimal and it's not a big deal, while other healthcare practitioners may tell you to avoid the tests completely. By now you have discovered that we don't believe in such "either-or" approaches. We believe in solutions that make sense. To us, it's not OK to say "Just don't worry about it," or "Just don't do it." We believe there is a better way. You can help protect the body from the harmful radiation before and after the test.

Taking antioxidants just before the test can give your cells added protection from the radiation exposure. While there are no clinical trials that prove protective benefit, there is solid theoretical rationale. Plus, there is little risk of harm and no danger of interfering with the scan. If you are taking any blood thinning or chemotherapy medications, consult with your doctor prior to adding these supplements—even for the short time that we are suggesting. Here is what we recommend.

Take at least three of the following nutrients three times each—approximately two hours prior to the scan, again within 30 minutes before the scan, and ideally within 30 minutes after the scan. These nutrients provide antioxidant support to help neutralize the radiation from the scans:

- Vitamin D = 1,000 IU each dose
- Vitamin E (mixed tocopherols only) = 400 IU each dose
- Glutathione (Setria® brand) = 250 mg each dose
- N-acetylcysteine = 250 mg each dose
- Alpha-lipoic acid = 100 mg each dose
- Spirulina or blue-green algae = 2,000 mg each dose
- Selenium citrate or picolinate = 100 mcg each dose *(Note: Two Brazil nuts provide the same amount of selenium)*

These nutrients have been shown to support the detoxification pathway and increase the body's antioxidant levels, thus helping to protect cells from damage. Rather than avoiding an important test, you can enhance your body's innate protective ability—it's the best of both worlds! In addition, pay careful attention to your diet and lifestyle, with a special focus on eating healthy, getting exercise, staying hydrated, and getting enough sleep.

is done to look for signs of infection, inflammation, and cancer of the bladder.

According to the American Cancer Society, beginning at age 30, women who have had three consecutive normal Pap test results can start doing screening every two to three years rather than annually. Women who are 70 years or older and have had at least three normal Pap tests in a row and no abnormal test results within the past 10 years may choose to stop having Pap tests.

Consult with your doctor if you are having any of the following symptoms:

- Unexplained pain in your lower belly or around the pelvic area
- Issues with your menstrual periods
- Vaginal discharge, itching, burning, or bad odor
- Severe cramps or other issues associated with premenstrual syndrome (PMS)
- Unexplained spotting after menopause

The major risk factor for cervical cancer is infection with certain strains of the human papillomavirus (HPV), a sexually transmitted virus. For this reason, testing for HPV during the pelvic exam in women who are sexually active is important. A key sign of HPV is genital warts. This is also the reason there is now a cervical cancer vaccine that helps prevent some HPV viruses. The use of this vaccine is becoming more widespread but remains controversial. We don't know the long-term risks of the vaccine, and we also know that it does not prevent all forms of HPV. While this vaccine can have some benefit to women and girls who are not receiving an annual Pap test, the best way to prevent cervical cancer remains with Pap test screening.

If cervical and uterine cancers are caught early, there is a great chance of a full recovery. If you have a family history of female cancers, discuss developing a proactive exam schedule with your doctor.

BREAST

You would think that breast cancer screening is pretty straightforward, but controversies exist here as well. Debate mostly involves timing and frequency of mammogram screening. A mammogram is an X-ray image of the breast, and digital mammography is the best type of mammogram.

The American Cancer Society recommends an annual mammogram beginning at age 40. Women who have a strong family history (mother or sister) of breast cancer or test positive for the BRCA gene should talk to their doctor about getting an MRI in addition to a mammogram. Breast ultrasound is another option for these women. High-risk women often ask our opinion on this matter. Women with a very strong family history of breast cancer (such as Karolyn's) and have tested positive for the BRCA gene, can consider doing a mammogram with an ultrasound every year and then a mammogram with an MRI every three years, as well as an annual physical that includes a clinical breast exam. These women should also do periodic self breast exams.

The American Cancer Society recommends women have a clinical breast exam (CBE), which is a breast exam done by a trained health-care professional, every three years between ages 20 and 39 and every year after age 40.

The controversy regarding mammography began in 2009 with the release of a new report by the U.S. Preventive Services Task Force. Based on published research, the task force recommends that women begin routine mammography at age 50, not age 40, and recommends a mammogram every two years until age 74 rather than annually. These recommendations are based upon their findings that the benefit of starting mammograms earlier and repeating them more often did not outweigh the harm they impose—mainly unnecessary biopsies and additional radiation exposure from the mammograms. The task force advised that women under age 50 should discuss the pros and cons of mammography with their physicians and that women at high risk may want to consider beginning mammography earlier than age 50. The task force also concluded that there is not enough evidence for them to recommend for or against mammography after age 74.

For those of you following this subject, you saw that the task force recommendation caused quite a stir in the national media.

Follow-up analyses in the medical literature have also opposed the task force's recommendation, suggesting that the benefits of early diagnosis from annual mammography beginning at age 40 outweigh its harm. In fact, according to research presented at the 2011 meeting of the American Society of Breast Surgeons, if women under the age of 50 are excluded from routine screening mammography, their risk of larger, more advanced tumors at diagnosis is increased, their recurrence rate increases six times, the likelihood of missing receptor-negative breast cancer (i.e., ER negative, PR negative, Her2-Neu negative) increases, and their odds for long-term survival are decreased. While we respect the conclusion of the task force and recognize that mammography does emit some radiation, can create false positive or negative results, and may cause women to undergo unnecessary and invasive procedures, which can be harmful to breast tissue, we believe the benefits of mammography outweigh its risks. It is important to discuss the frequency of mammography with your doctor, and beginning that discussion at the age of 40 (or earlier if you have risk factors) is appropriate. Mammography does detect some breast cancers and therefore remains a valuable tool. But it is just one tool. As mentioned previously, if you are concerned about breast cancer, discuss breast ultrasound and possibly MRI with your healthcare provider. This is especially important for women under age 50 who are at high risk, because younger women have a tendency to have more dense breast tissue and mammography is not as sensitive with dense tissue.

What about breast thermography? That's a question that we often hear as well. So far, there is not enough data to suggest that thermography can be used as a sole screening method for breast cancer. There is room for error in how the thermography is done, and the interpretation of the findings can vary. Until there is a certification program and guidelines for thermography testing, it should only be used in addition to standard screening. Once thermography standards and certification are developed, there may be a role for this minimally invasive imaging technique in the screening for breast cancer.

Promising screening and early diagnostic tests for breast cancer examine the blood or fluid expressed from the nipple (nipple aspirate) for elevated levels of markers associated with breast cancer.

With laboratory advances, these tests might create the opportunity to identify high-risk women for enhanced imaging surveillance, and provide additional rationale for implementing an aggressive risk-reduction program.

Another question that frequently pops up is, "What screening should I do if I've already had breast cancer?" This is a strategy that every breast cancer patient should discuss with her oncologist. A 2011 report in the *Journal of Surgical Oncology* concluded that in general, patients who are not experiencing any symptoms should receive an annual mammogram (or breast MRI if the original mammogram did not find the cancer), along with a physical examination by their doctor every three to four months for the first three years following treatment, every six months for the next two years, and then annually after five years. Additional scans and other tests may be recommended for patients who are experiencing symptoms.

Women at high risk for initial or recurrent breast cancer should be informed of these three options:

1. Rigorous breast surveillance using previously discussed screening (mammography, ultrasound, MRI, CBE)

2. Drug therapy, including anti-estrogenic agents

3. Prophylactic surgeries

A thorough discussion of these options as they relate to the person's individual risk, age, and quality of life issues should be discussed with their healthcare provider. In some cases prophylactic surgery may be a viable option; however, remember the number of people carrying the mutated gene is relatively small (about 10%). Discuss your options carefully before making your decision.

LUNG

Lung cancer is the most common cause of cancer death in both men and women worldwide. Lung cancer is most common in people who smoke, smoked regularly in the past, or have been exposed to significant second-hand smoke. People with a history of smoking or exposure to smokers, at minimum, need a chest X-ray annually. For nonsmokers, any persistent, dry cough should be evaluated with a chest X-ray. While chest X-rays are less expensive, they are also less accurate than a computed tomography (CT) test. An annual chest CT is the best screening tool, as it is more sensitive at finding lung tumors. Screening with CT scans reduces the rate of death from lung cancer by 20 percent. One of the problems with X-rays and CT scans is that these scans are not specific for lung cancer and find benign masses too. Researchers from Johns Hopkins University have been working on a solution to this problem. According to data presented at the American Association for Cancer Research in 2011, a blood test for a series of markers that are highly specific for non-small cell lung cancer (the most common type of lung cancer) shows promise in confirming or ruling out lung cancer after a CT scan. While more research is still needed, their hope is that this biomarker test will clarify the findings from lung CT.

KNOW YOUR BODY By Karolyn

My cancer diagnosis came less than three months after my mom died of advanced pancreatic cancer. Shockingly, the time between her diagnosis and her death was only three weeks. Her illness took a devastating toll on my family. She was our rock. So when I started experiencing shooting pain soon after she died, I told my sister that it was nothing. "I'm depressed," I said "and this is probably some psychological phantom pain related to mom's tumors." What I failed to mention was that these pains started before mom got sick. It wasn't until the pain doubled me over and became unbearable that I finally realized that this "phantom" wasn't going anywhere.

In hindsight, I should have paid more attention to the breakthrough bleeding, the fullness, weight gain, and bowel changes I was also experiencing. By the time I went to the doctor, I could even feel what would later be diagnosed as a cancerous tumor growing on the outside of my ovary and down my uterus. At the time (16 years ago), I was so lackadaisical about my health that I didn't even have a doctor, so I went to my sister's doctor for the diagnosis.

I have since learned my lesson. Proactive screening and regular checkups are a huge part of my cancer prevention program. I have also gotten to know my body better and can read the signals it sends me.

SKIN

Skin is one our most important and our largest organ. The two main layers of the skin are the dermis (lower) and epidermis (outer). Skin cancer begins in the epidermis and occurs in three basic types: basal cell carcinoma, squamous cell carcinoma, and melanoma. Basal cell is the most common and the easiest to treat, and melanoma is the most rare and difficult to treat.

The most effective way to screen for skin cancer is by examining the skin and paying close attention to any changes. If something looks abnormal, a biopsy may be required. Here are some key things to monitor:

- Moles that have changed in appearance
- Moles that have become larger
- Moles or spots that peel, bleed, or become itchy
- New moles, sores, or abnormal looking spots
- Ulcers or sores that do not heal

If you notice any of the above-mentioned changes, contact your doctor. The most important thing you can do to help prevent skin cancer is to get to know your skin and monitor any changes in collaboration with your doctor.

BEYOND CANCER SCREENING

Cancer screening is important, but to truly thrive, we need to go beyond cancer screening. We need to look at our bodies and our lives from head to toe. By keeping tabs on the following health areas, we will be staying in tune with our overall health and positively influencing all five pathways:

- Weight
- Mental health
- Vision
- Dental and gum health
- Heart health
- Bone density and joint health
- Weight

One of the biggest indicators that we are sliding down the slippery slope of poor health is weight gain. As you have heard us describe, carrying extra weight is a significant risk factor in the development of cancer, as well as other illnesses. Maintaining normal weight becomes a foundation for any cancer prevention plan. But what's even more important is that shedding those extra pounds will positively contribute to your quality of life as well.

Don't become obsessed with weighing yourself often, because the basic scale is not the most accurate judge of weight gain. BMI (as discussed on page 97) is more accurate. Newer scales include ways to measure your percentage of body fat, BMI, and weight. Also, simply pay close attention to how your clothes are fitting and how you physically feel. You can usually tell when you are starting to put on extra weight. It is normal to gain some weight as we age, particularly once we reach 50. This gradual and minimal weight gain is the result of the changing hormonal and metabolic state of our bodies. However, if your weight gain starts to accelerate to 5 to 10 pounds per decade, it is important to address it. Remember, accelerated weight gain (or surprisingly quick weight loss) should be discussed with your doctor. Don't let your weight fluctuations get out of hand. Call your doctor if you are concerned.

MENTAL HEALTH

Obesity is also associated with depression. Monitoring mental health is just as important as monitoring physical health. Depression, anxiety, inability to concentrate, and any other mental health issue should be addressed. These issues don't necessarily correlate with an increased risk for cancer, although people who are chronically depressed do not engage in healthful living and their physical health typically declines. The absence of healthy habits will, over time, increase the risk for cancer by impairing the health of the five key bodily pathways. In addition, monitoring your mental and emotional well-being is a way for you to remain present and engaged in your day-to-day life. And it is in the day-to-day where healthful habits are created and sustained.

VISION AND EYE HEALTH

As long as we are focused on the head right now, let's not forget about our eyes. As a part of your overall health plan, add an annual visit to the eye doctor. Not only is it important to evaluate the health of your eyes, but eye examinations can also detect certain signs of brain tumors. Vision is a wonderful gift and a sense that we can protect by following the Five to Thrive plan. That's right, the diet, lifestyle, and dietary supplements recommended will even enhance the health of your eyes. Some of those colorful fruits and vegetables have compounds that have an affinity to the eyes and can protect and benefit eye health.

In addition to adding more color to your diet, you may want to consider these tips for eye health:

- Use only all-natural eye drops

- Stay well hydrated

- Get enough sleep

- Take breaks from computer work

- Wear sunglasses when outdoors, to protect eyes not only from sun glare but also from wind

DENTAL AND GUM HEALTH

Regular dental checkups are critical to help screen for head and neck cancers and cancers in the mouth; however, that's just the beginning. The health of your mouth can reflect the health of your entire body. If you think about it, gum disease is an inflammatory condition. If our gums are inflamed, could we have chronic inflammation elsewhere? Something seemingly as benign as bad breath can indicate other issues, such as gastrointestinal disorders, a respiratory infection, or even diabetes.

If you are going to have a proactive plan to prevent cancer, you need to include regular visits to the dentist. In addition, consistent, effective oral health care that includes meticulous brush-

COMPLETELY OUT OF THE BLUE!

By Dr. Alschuler

At the age of 41 and in apparent good health, I went to my annual checkup expecting the usual clean bill of health. During the breast examination, my very astute gynecologist told me that she felt a lump that she did not remember being there before. She was not worried, but thought it would be a good idea for me to get a mammogram, "just to be sure." I thought that sounded like a good idea, especially since I was positive that I did not have cancer.

Because of my age, my breast tissue was too dense for the mammogram to find anything, so I had a breast ultrasound. The ultrasound showed the lump, and it looked benign. I was given two options, come back in six months to re-check the lump for changes via ultrasound or come back next week for an ultrasound guided needle biopsy. I left the appointment feeling relieved that I did not have to go back for another 6 months. Fortunately, I had a very astute and caring partner who suggested that I not take the risk of missing something and encouraged me to get the biopsy. Boy, am I glad I did! Despite the radiologist's comment during the biopsy, "I am 99 percent sure that this is not cancer," it was.

That is how my personal odyssey into the world of cancer started. After much treatment and many breast MRIs later, I am now without evidence of breast cancer. I can say that I am very, very grateful that I paid enough attention to my health, despite feeling healthy, to get my annual examination and the screening tests that followed.

---

ing and flossing is essential. If you have issues with gum disease, we recommend supplemental CoQ10 (Kyolic Formula 110) at a dose of 60–100 mg daily and even an all-natural rinse that contains CoQ10.

Your mouth is the first entry point in the digestion pathway. In addition to giving us the pleasure of taste, a lot of activity takes place in that important foyer to the rest of your body. Keeping your mouth healthy will contribute to your quality of life in a big way.

HEART HEALTH

Heart disease is the leading cause of death in the United States—accounting for more than one in four deaths of Americans. Almost one-third of all deaths globally are attributed to heart disease and stroke. Protecting your heart is a cornerstone of any health-enhancing program.

Screening for high blood pressure and high cholesterol are important during your annual checkup. It is also critical to discuss any family history with your doctor. It is important to be on the lookout for the following symptoms of heart disease, and be sure to talk with your doctor about them:

- Heart palpitations (skipping, irregular, faster heartbeat)
- Feeling of fullness and frequent indigestion
- Extreme fatigue, weakness, or anxiety
- Long-standing chest discomfort or pain
- Unexplained headaches, especially in the morning
- Cold or dusky colored hands or feet
- Unexplained weight gain with swelling in one or both feet

As expected, the heart will also thrive on the Five to Thrive plan. The heart depends upon a diet of colorful fruits and vegetables, consistent physical activity, love, joy, and the many other aspects that we emphasize.

BONE HEALTH

While the heart is the pump that keeps us moving, it's the health of our bones that helps us to be active, strong, and vibrant. Osteopenia and osteoporosis are conditions characterized by thin, fragile bones. A bone density test can help monitor the bone health. Typically, all men and women should undergo bone density tests beginning at the age of 65. However, certain risk factors may indicate the need to start this screening earlier so discuss this with your doctor. The following put you at greater risk for osteoporosis:

- Family history of osteoporosis
- Previous history of having received chemotherapy, long-term (greater than 3 months) steroid use, or radiation therapy to the spine or hips
- Surgically induced menopause
- Excessive thinness
- Sedentary lifestyle
- History of smoking
- Nutrient deficiencies (e.g., calcium, vitamin D, vitamin K, boron, strontium)
- History of consuming more than two alcoholic drinks daily for women and more than three alcoholic drinks daily for men

A cost-effective initial screening test to take a first look at bone density is a noninvasive ultrasound of the heel bone. If this test is abnormal, a more accurate screening test is next. Bone density is best determined with a noninvasive test called a DEXA (dual energy X-ray absorptiometry). This 10-minute test accurately assesses the extent of any bone loss. The results of a DEXA scan guide therapy choices. While medications such as bisphosphonate drugs are sometimes indicated, there are also viable natural strategies that may reduce or eliminate the need for these drugs, especially in the earlier stages of osteoporosis.

So to recap, beyond cancer screening, we need to have a "head to toe" attitude about our general health. This includes keeping tabs on our weight, being honest about our mental health, seeing the eye doctor on a regular basis, visiting the dentist consistently, making sure our heart is pumping strong, and checking on and supporting our bone density. Seems simple enough!

THE FUTURE

Effective cancer screening tests are presently available, but what can we expect in the future? Following are some promising opportunities on the horizon, but it remains to be seen if they will come to fruition in terms of effective screening.

Circulating tumor cells. Circulating tumor cell (CTC) tests capture cancer cells that are circulating in the blood. These cells can then be analyzed chemically and microscopically. This analysis can provide useful information about the nature of the cancer, identify potential targets for therapies, and may even give prognostic information. Some oncologists utilize these tests to help them learn about the molecular characteristics of an individual's cancer, which, in turn, helps determine their selection of therapies. These tests are still being studied, so they are not yet widely used. However, they offer a very promising way to learn about the state of someone's cancer with a simple blood draw. CTCs are present in people with metastatic cancer and can also be found in the blood of people with early-stage cancers. For instance, people who have received chemotherapy for early-stage breast cancer and who have CTCs after treatment have reduced survival rates. This is because circulating tumor cells have the potential to seed secondary tumors in other parts of the body. Knowing about the presence of CTCs after what is presumed to be definitive treatment creates the opportunity for additional (and different) treatment at a time when it really counts. The newer generation of the CTC test is much better at catching the tumor cells and also catches what appear to be microclusters of CTCs. These groupings of cancer cells may be directly implicated in metastasis. We are sure we will be hearing more about CTCs in the future, as this will likely become an increasingly important component of cancer care and may also have implications in screening.

More sophisticated molecular genetic testing. Genetic testing, our support of patients receiving genetic testing, and confirmation of the benefits of genetic testing is still in its infancy. However, research continues to progress in this area. For example, research published in *Cancer Prevention Research* may have uncovered a new risk factor for developing breast cancer—DNA methylation modifications to the BRCA1 gene—before it can be detected as being mutated. BRCA1 is a DNA-repair gene and methylation is the epigenetic way of silencing its activity. A test that determines the methylation state of this gene will give us not only a window into the risk for cancer development, but also an opportunity to implement the lifestyle strategies included in this Five to Thrive prevention plan to change the epigenetic influences on this gene.

Another promising area of detection is with genetic testing. For instance, in 2007 researchers from Johns Hopkins published data in the *American Journal of Obstetrics & Gynecology* showing that a screening test can detect mutations of the TP53 gene, which is associated with more aggressive, harder-to-treat ovarian cancers. The researchers note that the present options for ovarian cancer screening have limited use, and research in the area of ovarian cancer screening is needed.

BEING PROACTIVE

Achieving cancer prevention success requires a shift in perspective. From the book *The Art of Possibility*, Rosamund Stone Zander and Benjamin Zander write, "Life often looks like an obstacle course. In order to maximize success, we spend a good deal of time discussing what stands in the way of it." Let's not look at results from a screening test as a roadblock standing in the way of our happiness. Rather, let's look at it as information that will help us navigate the obstacle course of life. Keep your eye on the prize—thriving!

 **HIGH FIVE TIP** *Keep a separate health calendar that keeps track of when you are due to see your doctors, including your eye doctor and your dentist. Also pay close attention to how your body is responding to life on a daily basis. Getting to know your body from head to toe is critical so you can then share any new information with your doctors. Remember, you are in charge!*

CHAPTER

SERVICE, SPIRIT, AND **SOUL**

We sat transfixed in the second row of an auditorium filled with more than 900 people, mostly healthcare professionals, as integrative healthcare icon Rachel Naomi Remen, MD, walked on stage. Her topic: Integrating the spirit into healthcare. Her philosophy: Fixing is the work of the ego, but service is the work of the soul.

"When you help, you see life as weak. When you fix, you see life as broken. When you serve, you see life as whole," she explained. Rachel has inspired our work and our journey. And her message of service, spirit, and soul coincides strongly with what we believe and promote in our cancer work.

As we discussed in Chapter 6, there are ways to rejuvenate your physical, emotional, and even cellular health. In this chapter we shed light on the final dimension and the most significant aspects of

ARE YOU A CONTRIBUTION?

We view service as a frame of mind, a way of being. It's more of a mentality than one specific act. In the enlightening book *The Art of Possibility*, husband and wife team Rosamund and Benjamin Zander provide practical ways we can invite fulfillment into our human experience. The chapter "Being a Contribution" points out that life can be inspired from a place of contribution rather than the domain of success: "Naming oneself and others as a contribution produces a shift away from self-concern and engages us in a relationship with others that is an arena for making a difference." Not just making a difference, we would add, but truly thriving as you experience a vital and fulfilled life. Ask yourself this today: How will you be a *contribution* this week?

deep rejuvenation. Valuing service, nurturing spirit, and connecting with the authentic soul that thrives within and around us is the fabric of our existence. This is the foundation of our very being, leading us to meaning, fulfillment, and thriving in the most ultimate sense.

OUR ROOTS RUN DEEP

Some people are fascinated with genealogy—discovering their family history in hopes of unlocking the mystery of who they are and why they are here. Yes, genealogy can be intriguing; and yet most of us have heard the stories of twins separated at birth only to grow up as two very different people even though they have identical genetics. Our roots can influence who we are, but they are only part of the story.

For example, let's consider the two of us. We grew up in completely different settings: one from highly educated parents in a small family, the other one of six children from blue-collar beginnings. Somewhat predictably, one of us took the road of higher learning while the other became an entrepreneur. We both value hard work, but that work manifests itself differently. One becomes a doctor, the other a writer. And here is where our paths become far more similar than dissimilar.

While our roots and our upbringing were different, we became adults with the same vision for our lives—to satisfy our voracious appetites for information and to distill and dispense that information. And yet, that is still not what cemented our bond. As daughters of a parent who died of pancreatic cancer and as previous cancer patients ourselves, we share something even more powerful than genes—we have experiences that connect our souls. Who would have predicted that we would be here—sharing our vision, creating together, and nurturing this friendship? Perhaps even before we knew it, our souls were communicating and we were destined to do this work together. Who knows? What we do know is that it's vital to infuse service, soul, and spirit into the epigenetic mix of influencers when it comes to living a vital life.

When we embarked on this journey together more than a decade ago, we did not know where it would take us. But here we are. These

LET THERE BE LIGHT

A story from Rachel Naomi Remen, MD

In the process of recovering from kidney cancer, one of my patients underwent a transformation from a hard-driving CEO to a volunteer and supporter of many good causes. He told me of the experience, which had changed his way of moving through the world. As a child of atheistic and intellectual parents, he had no religious upbringing or spiritual inclination and had immersed himself in the world of competition and business with much success. Although his business had formerly been the focus of his life, his cancer and its treatment now required him to be away from the multitasking demands and pressures of his work and instead to spend several months in the quiet of his living room.

At first this had been frightening and deeply disorienting, but then as the fatigue of his chemotherapy took hold, he had simply surrendered to the silence and spent hours on his couch dozing in the company of his cat. One afternoon as he lay drifting in and out of sleep, he found himself looking at a bookshelf on the opposite wall. It seemed to him that one of the books stood out from the others in an odd way. Getting up for a closer look he saw that it was the very same Bible that the clergyman who had performed his marriage years ago had given to him and his wife. Taking it back to the couch he opened it for the first time and started to read the story of the beginning of the world. He was surprised to feel a deep response to the simple words, how real and familiar and terrifying the formlessness and darkness felt to him and how it seemed to be somehow connected to the terrible recent events in his life. And then he encountered the statement with which the world begins: "Let there be light." He lay there for a time feeling the great power in these four words wash over him.

As he ruminated about this, the words suddenly shifted their meaning, and he realized that they were addressed to him personally—that he personally was able to choose to act in ways that increased the light in the world. He had never considered this possibility before, but over the next days and weeks it became a more and more compelling thought, until he recognized it as a deep yearning in himself to live in a certain way. That perhaps the purpose of life was not to become wealthy or succeed in business or to leave a financial inheritance to his children as he had thought. Perhaps he might have the chance to fulfill the real purpose of life and bring more light into the world. Perhaps this was the inheritance he could leave to his children.

three guiding principles—service, soul, spirit—have transformed our journey, and we'd like to show you how they can influence your path and your ability to thrive. First, let's explore the gift of service.

PAY IT FORWARD

We often hear people say, "I've never done any volunteer work, so I'm just not sure how best I can serve." Remember our conversation about exercise and shifting your thinking from spandex and mirrors to gardening and dancing? The same is true for service—if you look

THE HUMBLE SOUL OF SERVICE

By Dr. Alschuler

Ann, a successful business owner, attorney, and nurse is wearing a shirt with "Be in Gratitude" printed on it. It is her after-hours comfortable shirt that is perfect as she is collecting trash from throughout the house to add to the big outdoor can. Finishing the trash collection, she takes her iced tea up to the guest bedroom where she has her ironing board set up. As she irons, she plans out when she can best fit in a needed trip to the grocery store. Later, sitting on the couch to watch a bit of television, she asks her partner how the day went and if there was anything to be added to the grocery list. A few more items are tacked on. The evening comes to a close and they retire for the night.

These household chores, the mundane day-to-day tasks that Ann does without complaint or resentment are, perhaps, the ultimate form of service. With every shirt ironed, piece of trash collected, or trip to the grocery store, Ann expresses her love and gratitude for her partner and their life together. Without glory or grand finales, Ann simply keeps on giving. "Work done in the spirit of service is worship," from the Baha'i teachings, is exactly what Ann's chores are. Worship is defined as a feeling of adoring reverence or regard. Each chore that Ann does expresses her willingness to expend some of her life force for the good of another. Each act confirms her connection to life and especially to her loved one. By being a contribution, Ann transforms the mundane into a powerful expression of her spirit, a spirit dominated by generosity. The gratitude that she hears from her partner is gratitude not just for the wrinkle-free clothes, but also for Ann's gracious and tender presence in the world.

at it differently, you'll find ways it fits. What's more, there is scientific evidence that service can promote your health.

Scientific studies show those who serve in the traditional sense of volunteering their time and energy have enhanced physical and mental health. A 2007 comprehensive report by the Corporation for National & Community Service reviewed 30 different studies that looked at how volunteering affected health. The researchers found that volunteers, especially older people, lived longer and had lower rates of both depression and heart disease compared to those who did not volunteer.

How can serving others help your health? This is certainly a new area of study, but one thought is that our need to help is fundamental and when we deny it, we deny an important part of who we are. From a physiological epigenetic standpoint, preliminary research shows there is a "helper's high" that produces oxytocin, a brain neurotransmitter that is associated with bonding, trust, and generosity. While there is still a lot to learn about oxytocin, its release can be health-promoting. Preliminary animal and human data show that oxytocin release can enhance immunity and reduce inflammation, while oxytocin suppression may do just the opposite.

So helping others not only makes us happier, it can make us healthier. But does that mean we have to carve out time in an already busy schedule to volunteer in our communities? Not necessarily. While we both value the act of service in the form of volunteering, the idea of service goes beyond that initial definition. To us, service is more than something we do once a month or even once a week. Service is a frame of mind, a way of thinking, a way of being. Service is less about structure and more about substance—our substance as a human race—and how we conduct ourselves in every moment of every day.

Abraham Maslow, PhD, famed psychology professor and one of the pioneers of the Human Potential Movement, once said that if all you have is a hammer, everything will begin to look like a nail. While Maslow wasn't talking about service, he was saying that it's important to broaden our view and look at things differently—

this includes our perception of what it means to serve. The act of service can be accomplished in many different ways, and the best acts of service are unexpected, frequent, and heartfelt.

Do you recall the 2000 movie *Pay it Forward* starring Kevin Spacey, Helen Hunt, and Haley Joel Osment? In the movie, the child (Haley Joel) is given the assignment of finding a way to change the world. He does this by developing and implementing a concept that involves doing something good for someone when something good is done for you. You don't "pay it back" by doing something good for the person who did something good for you; you "pay it forward" by doing something totally unexpected and kind for someone else, someone new. In the movie, a chain reaction of good deeds is created.

HORSES IN HEAVEN By Karolyn

I think the concept of dreaming is a bit odd. Dreams have so many dimensions—scary, funny, warm, weird. But my favorite dream is the one I had about a year after my mom died.

My mom and I had always been avid horseback riders. It was something we shared since I was 7, and those were times I thoroughly cherished. But then my mom had a horseback riding injury that broke her back. She was told she would never ride again. She did, in fact, ride a horse again, but she was nearly always in pain. In hindsight, her pancreatic cancer most likely contributed to her back pain.

In the dream, she gallops to me riding a beautiful white horse. I remember in the dream thinking that was odd because my mom always loved black horses (funny how even in our dreams we can get distracted by details). She spins to a stop in front of me—I am of course on horseback as well—and says, "Did you see that? Wasn't that amazing? I can ride again, and it's so much fun!" With that she gave me one of her mischievous crooked smiles, turned her horse quickly, and ran off in the distance. I chased after her but woke up before I caught up.

Was this dream a figment of my imagination, my desire to want her to be out of pain, horseback riding in heaven? Who knows, but I don't care. I think of that dream often and I'm sure I will continue to think of it until the day I'm riding horses again with her.

To have a service mentality is to continually practice unexpected acts of kindness regardless of what you receive in return. For example, a nice gesture is serving your partner breakfast in bed on his birthday, but what would happen if you served him breakfast in bed unexpectedly on a random Saturday? And it's not just the act of serving him breakfast. What if you had a hand written note on the tray and then enjoyed breakfast with him in bed as you told him how much you appreciated him? You see, service is not in just what we do; it's in what we say, and even what we think and feel. Seeing goodness in others and expressing that appreciation is an act of service that is priceless.

Rachel says it so eloquently, "When we serve, we see the unborn wholeness in others; we collaborate with it and strengthen it. Others may then be able to see their wholeness for themselves for the first time."

CONNECTION IS CRITICAL

One aspect we love about service is the connection it creates. Having a service attitude connects us with others. This is confirmed in the scientific literature: Studies show that people who serve feel less isolated and more connected. Why is connection so critical?

University of Houston research professor and renowned speaker Brené Brown, PhD, LMSW, says connection is important because it's how we are neurobiologically "wired." Connection is "what gives purpose and meaning to our lives. It's why we're here." In her acclaimed talk on the topic of vulnerability, Brown explained that in order for true connection to take place, we must let ourselves be seen. This is the essence of vulnerability. Perhaps you've thought of vulnerability as a negative, a sign of weakness, but nothing could be further from the truth. Vulnerability is the gateway to true connection.

But to be vulnerable we need two key ingredients: the courage to be authentic and compassion for others. We discussed the importance of authenticity in Chapter 3. Compassion involves understanding that our actions affect our health and our lives. Our actions also impact and are impacted by others. Compassion also gives us great leniency with others as we allow them to be imperfect, make mistakes, and have idiosyncrasies. Our expectations for others and for ourselves are replaced with gratitude for simply being who we each grandly are. With this realization, we can experience true, rewarding connection—with ourselves, others, and our own bodies.

Yes, there is a connection between mind, body, and spirit. In fact, it is this interplay, this interconnectedness of mind, body, and spirit that can deeply influence the five key pathways. While this area of study is still a twinkle in the eyes of some of today's most forward thinkers, we ask this question: What if our thoughts do in fact play a significant role in how our bodies feel and how illness or wellness develops? One thing is for sure: There are no negative side effects of thinking positively, connecting with others, and being kind.

Which brings us to a conversation about soul. There is soul food, soul music, and even soul mates, but what about the soul of a thriver? How do we get in touch with that soul?

THE SOUL OF A THRIVER

The term soul is sometimes used interchangeably with the word spirit, but we see them as two different things. Spirit is a vital force that motivates, radiates, and permeates our being. Soul is the fundamental essence of who we are—transcending the physical and embracing the multidimensional.

The terms "spirit" and "soul" can have varying religious connotations. In some religious practice, the soul is life and subject to death, but the spirit can live on forever. Other religions believe the soul is what lives on forever. Some religions believe the soul can be reincarnated, while others believe death is the end of the existence of both spirit and soul. Our intention is not to have a religious debate or even discuss religion at all. We don't view spirit or soul as religious; we view them as ways of being and experiencing a vital existence.

THE SOULFUL LIFE OF AN OCCASIONALLY DITZY BLONDE

By Dr. Alschuler

My sister, Britt, has a collection of stories about me— about my more absentminded moments, to be exact—that she has archived as "Lise's ditzy blond moments." Over the years, as we have shared some good belly laughs over my mishaps, she has surreptitiously committed them to memory. She has quite a library by now and pulls one out every now then. In fact, I suspect that there are quite a few people in her life who would only recognize me by a rendition of these events.

She might tell a story about me giving a complicated lecture to an audience of healthcare professionals to many accolades only to be followed by my leaving the lecture to go to my car, and forgetting completely where my car was parked. After an hour of trolling the garage, I finally happened upon it. Then there was the time I grabbed the Lysol deodorizer can from the bathroom by mistake and walked through the office clutching it along with my note pad, oblivious to the stares of my coworkers, before finally realizing that I was still carrying the can. I could go on and on, but I will stop here.

The point of sharing these stories is to demonstrate the naked and whole truth of living a soulful life. Existing alongside my intellectual accomplishments are my clumsy mishaps. My clinical insights share space with my feelings of utter bewilderment at the simplest things. I, just like every other human being, am a blend of contradictions and imperfections. It is the courage to accept these inconsistencies and faults that gives my soul room to breathe in the spirit of life.

Soul is not something we have; it is who we are. You have a body but you are a soul. Motivational speaker and author Wayne Dyer says it this way, "Begin to see yourself as a soul with a body rather than a body with a soul." The soul is the moral, emotional, and spiritual personification of our potential.

By now you've come to know that we are pragmatic authors. While we love entertaining thoughts of our life force, we also want practical ways to invite more *soul* into our lives. We've come up with these five (yes five!) characteristics of the soul of a thriver:

1. **Not a pretender.** Sometimes it can be easy to become someone we are not, or to slip into a routine where we pretend that there are no ramifications for our actions. The soul of a thriver is authentic to their essence and has no compulsion to be anyone or anything different.

2. **Fearless.** The soul of a thriver is not afraid to be vulnerable and to shine a light on all aspects of his character. Being fearless does not mean we are never afraid. It means we acknowledge our fears and take the next step directly into them. A thriver is bold, daring, and courageous.

3. **Embraces uncertainty.** In her talk, Brown says there is such a tendency to make everything uncertain certain. "I'm right, you're wrong, shut up," she exclaims. By embracing uncertainty, the soul of a thriver is open to the possibilities that each moment holds.

4. **Expansive.** The soul of the thriver welcomes an ever-expanding perception of everything. The soul listens, is aware, and is receptive.

5. **Spirit-filled.** Spirit is the spark that keeps our soul's flame lit. Spirit saturates human existence, and the soul of a thriver seeks this depth to connect with other beings.

To embrace the characteristics of the soul of a thriver is to honor the prevailing spirit surrounding us.

THE SPIRIT WITHIN AND AROUND

Famous author Stephen Covey wrote, "We are not human beings on a spiritual journey. We are spiritual beings on a human journey." Similar to Dyer's view of the soul, we are deeply aware that we are more than a physical body.

To be spiritual infuses religion, but can also transcend it. A spiritual life is one lived with acute awareness and genuine openness. Spirit is the fire in our belly, the life force that propels us into existence. Being attuned to the spirited side of life requires us to be present and engaged. Here are some ways to gain a greater sense of our spiritual life. Consider these examples:

1. **Birth:** Watching the birth of another living being (animal or human) allows us to bear witness to the beginning of the potential embodied in the newborn before us.

2. **Death:** Witnessing death allows us a touch point with the unguarded, naked transition from embodied life to purely spirit life.

3. **Nature:** The expansiveness of the mountains, power of lakes and streams, and serenity of trees and flowers sparks the flame of our spirituality, awe, and wonder.

4. **Silence:** Experiencing silence or allowing ourselves to listen to the natural sounds around us can be brought out in forms of meditation, yoga, and other contemplative spiritual activities. Within silence, we can find undistracted bliss.

5. **Interaction:** Appreciating the interactions we have with a child, a family pet, or a close friend instills appreciation that ignites our spiritual sense.

Spirituality is personal and individual. For this reason, a hallmark of the spiritual thriver is to be nonjudgmental of the spiritual practices of others. It is our right to embrace our spirituality, but it is not our right to judge how others explore their spirituality. The key is not to have the "right" spiritual practice; it is to be fully open to the fact that you are a spiritual being. Embracing your spiritual nature will help instill in you a sense of peace, contentment, and fulfillment.

PUTTING IT ALL TOGETHER

We are spiritual, soul-filled beings with a unique and vital ability to connect and serve. We are multidimensional, complex creatures; however, embracing service, soul, and spirit can be as simple

DON'T WORRY ABOUT ME

By Karolyn

I was brought up strict Catholic. As a child, I was taught the rosary, went to the confessional, and performed the other rituals associated with the religion. As an adult, I realized that my strict upbringing was about believing in a higher power. My mom loved the rituals, the prayers, and her faith. But in the last days of her physical life, she told me that it wasn't the *religion* she loved because that's "mostly manmade." She loved the fact that her faith gave her a compass to live by, and it also gave her something bigger to believe in. It was her faith that caused her to ask her sister to come to her in a dream after she passed, and it was my faith that asked the same question of my mom as she waited to make her transition. "I'll try," she said sheepishly. I think she believed she could, but she wasn't about to make any guarantees.

It was Christmas time when she was sick. Fortunately, she was able to remain at home. When she needed something, she rang Christmas bells, and one of us would come running. Toward the end of her time, there was one night when I was on "duty" as I dozed nearby. At about 2 a.m. I heard the bells ring and sprang into action. I stood by her bed and asked, "What is it mom? What do you need?" She said, "Sit down." At first I must admit that I was a bit irritated that she didn't need anything at all and really just wanted to talk. I sat beside her as I rubbed the sleep from my eyes.

"Don't worry about me," she began. Impatiently, and inaccurately I might add, I said, "Mom I'm not worried." "No, really, I mean it, don't worry about me." She paused because she knew she had my attention. "He's already here with me at night, and he said he will bring me there himself." Her words took my breath away because it reminded me of the magnitude of it all. But then I was oddly at peace. "I'm so glad to hear that mom," I said as I held her hand. I was comforted.

My mom gave me a gift of infinite value—the gift of spirit.

as wrapping yourself in a warm blanket on a cool night—it can become second nature.

In this book we have covered a great deal of ground. We have:

- exposed you to the fascinating and growing field of epigenetics and the fact that we can influence how our genes behave;

- described the five key pathways and why they are so important to cancer prevention;

- introduced ways to encourage more love, laughter, and joy into your life;

- discussed the importance of movement and diet;

- explained how you can rejuvenate your mind, body, and spirit;

- clarified the confusing world of dietary supplements;

- emphasized the importance of regular check-ups and getting in tune with your body; and

- explored what it can look like to have the spirit of a thriver.

What's next? Well, it's time to THRIVE of course!

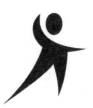 **HIGH FIVE TIP** *Imagine lying in lush, freshly cut grass on a warm summer's day. The smell of fresh air is intoxicating as you feel the sun on your skin, the tickle of the grass in your hands, and the weight of your body touching the earth. This represents spirit to us. How do you visually describe spirit? Take a moment to think about—or even better, write about—what causes you to feel spirit in your life. What does that look and feel like? Take your time and have fun with this.*

RESOURCES

Following is a list of books, organizations, manufacturers, and websites that can provide additional valuable health information. Please keep in mind, this is not meant to be an exhaustive list, however, it does represent some of our favorites.

BOOKS

Inspirational

Kitchen Table Wisdom and *My Grandfather's Blessings* both by Rachel Naomi Remen, MD

The Art of Possibility: Transforming Professional and Personal Life by Rosamund Stone Zander and Benjamin Zander

The Chemistry of Joy and *The Chemistry of Calm* both by Henry Emmons, MD

The Power of Now by Eckhart Tolle

When Things Fall Apart by Pema Chodron

Why I Wake Early by Mary Oliver

Health

8 Weeks of Women's Wellness by Marianne Marchese, ND

Definitive Guide to Cancer by Lise Alschuler, ND, and Karolyn A. Gazella

Healing Depression by Peter Bongiorno, ND, LAc

How to Talk With Your Doctor by Ronald L. Hoffman, MD

Life Over Cancer by Keith Block, MD

One Bite at a Time: Nourishing Recipes for Cancer Survivors and Their Friends by Rebecca Katz and Mat Edelson

The Encyclopedia of Healing Foods by Michael Murray, ND

The Seven Levels of Healing by Jeremy Geffen, MD

Unstuck: Your Guide to the Seven-Stage Journey out of Depression by James S. Gordon, MD

What the Drug Companies Won't Tell you and Your Doctor Doesn't Know by Michael Murray, ND

OTHER HEALTH BOOKS AND MAGAZINES PUBLISHED BY ACTIVE INTEREST MEDIA

Boost Your Health with Bacteria by Fred Pescatore, MD, and Karolyn A. Gazella

Living Lessons: My Journey of Faith, Love, and Cutting-Edge Cancer Therapy by Mark Shigihara, RPh, and Kim Erickson

Whole Body Cleansing by Gaetano Morello, ND

Amazing Wellness magazine (www.amazingwellnessmag.com)

Better Nutrition magazine (www.betternutrition.com)

Vegetarian Times (www.vegetariantimes.com)

Yoga Journal (www.yogajournal.com)

ORGANIZATIONS

American Academy of Environmental Medicine (www.aaemonline.org)

American Association of Naturopathic Physicians (www.naturopathic.org)

Oncology Association of Naturopathic Physicians (www.oncanp.org)

American Holistic Medical Association (www.holisticmedicine.org)

National Center for Homeopathy (www.homeopathic.org)

Society for Integrative Oncology (www.integrativeonc.org)

PRODUCTS MENTIONED

EuroPharma

866-598-5487

Founded by natural health pioneer Terry Lemerond, EuroPharma, Inc., is the maker of the retail brand, *Terry Naturally*, and the health practitioner brand, EuroMedica. Both product lines provide clinically proven dietary supplements to natural health stores and healthcare professionals. Some of their unique products include Curamin for pain and CuraMed, both of which include BCM-95® high absorption curcumin, and the omega 3 product, Vectomega. For more information, visit www.europharmausa.com. Health practitioners can also visit the EuroMedica website at www.euromedicausa.com.

Kyowa Hakko USA

212-319-5353

Kyowa Hakko Bio is an international health ingredients manufacturer and world leader in the development, manufacturing, and marketing of pharmaceuticals, nutraceuticals, and food products. Kyowa Hakko U.S.A., Inc. (Kyowa Hakko USA) is a wholly owned subsidiary of Kyowa Hakko Bio Co., Ltd., headquartered in Tokyo, Japan. Kyowa Hakko is the maker of branded ingredients including Cognizin® Citicoline, Hydrafend™ Hyaluronic Acid, Lumistor® L-Hydroxyproline, Setria® Glutathione, Pantein® PantothenicAcid, Kyowa CoQ10®, and Sustamine™ L-Alanyl-LGlutamine. Visit www.kyowa-usa.com, www.setriaglutathione.com, www.cognizin.com, www.sustamine.com or www.pantesin.com for additional information.

Taiyo International

763-398-3003

Taiyo is a leading manufacturer of functional ingredients for the food, beverage, and supplement industries. Taiyo focuses on the development of innovative ingredients, derived from natural sources, to further develop the body's ability to protect and manage one's health. Products include Suntheanine® (unique amino acid which reduces stress and improves focus without drowsiness), Sunphenon® (full range of green tea catechins), Matcha Powder (natural green tea leaf), SunActive® series, including iron, zinc, CoQ10, and Sunfiber®, a True Regulating galactomannan soluble dietary fiber. For more information visit www.taiyointernational.com.

Wakunaga

800-421-2998

Established almost 40 years ago, Wakunaga is a leader in scientific research and state-of-the-art manufacturing. They are best known for their line of supplements that feature a unique aged garlic extract known as Kyolic. They offer a full line of products available to both natural health stores and healthcare professionals. For more information visit www.kyolic.com.

OTHER ONLINE RESOURCES

Lise Alschuler, ND, FABNO
(www.drlise.net)

Commonweal Health and Environmental Research Institute
(www.commonweal.org)

Emerson Ecologics
(www.emersonecologics.com)

EmobodiWorks
(www.embodiworks.org)

Five2Thrive
(www.Five2Thrive.com)

Karolyn A. Gazella
(www.karolyngazella.com)

Natural Medicine Journal
(www.naturalmedicinejournal.com)

FITNESS ASSESSMENT

There are some excellent fitness assessment and tracking programs online, most of which are also available as apps for smart phones. These applications assist the user in creating and monitoring individualized diet and exercise plans based upon their current weight, activity level, and goals.

Some of our favorites are:
www.myfitnesspal.com
www.sparkpeople.com
www.fitday.com
www.caloriecount.com

REFERENCES BY CHAPTER

INTRODUCTION

Alschuler L, Gazella K. *The Definitive Guide to Cancer 3rd Edition* (Random House 2010).

Mariotto AB, et al. Projections of the cost of cancer care in the United States: 2010–2020. *J Natl Cancer Inst.* 2011;103(2):117-128.

Niederdeppe J, Levy AG. Fatalistic beliefs about cancer prevention and three prevention behaviors. *Cancer Epidemiol Biomarkers Prev.* 2007;16(5):998-1003.

Zimmerman GL, Olsen CG, Bosworth MF. A 'stage of change' approach to helping patients change behavior. *Am Fam Physician GP.* 2000;61:1409-1416.

CHAPTER 2

Ghadirian P, Narod S, Fafard E, Costa M, Robidoux A, Nkondjock A. Breast cancer risk in relation to the joint effect of BRCA mutations and diet diversity. *Breast Cancer Res Treat.* 2009;117(2):417-422.

Nkondjock A, Robidoux A, Paredes Y, Narod SA, Ghadirian P. Diet, lifestyle and BRCA-related breast cancer risk among French-Canadians. *Breast Cancer Res Treat.* 2006;98(3):285-294.

Ornish D, Lin J, Daubenmier J, et al. Increased telomerase activity and comprehensive lifestyle changes: a pilot study. *Lancet Oncol.* 2008; 9(11):1048-1057.

CHAPTER 3

"Yoga Philosophy—Namaste." Yoga Heals Us. Available at: http://yogahealsus.com/about3.html. Accessed May 22, 2011.

Christie W, Moore C. The impact of humor on patients with cancer. *Clin J Oncol Nurs.* 2005;9(2):211-218.

Costanzo ES, et al. Psychosocial factors and interleukin-6 among women and advanced ovarian cancer. *Cancer.* 2005;104:305-313.

Danner DD, Snowdon DA, Friesen WV. Positive emotions in early life and longevity: finding from the nun study. *J Pers Soc Psychol.* 2001;80(5):804-813.

DeMoor JS, et al. Optimism, distress, health-related quality of life, and change in cancer antigen 125 among patients with ovarian cancer undergoing chemotherapy. *Psychosomatic Medicine.* 2006;68:555-562.

Hershberger PJ. Prescribing happiness: Positive psychology and family medicine. *Fam Med.* 2005;37(9):630-634.

Holman EA, et al. Terrorism, acute stress, and cardiovascular health. A 3-year national study following the September 11th attacks. *Arch Gen Psychiatr.* 2008;65(1):73-80.

Phillips AC, et al. Bereavement and marriage are associated with antibody response to influenza vaccination in the elderly. *Brain Behav Immun.* 2006;20(3):279-289.

Ram D. *Grist for the Mill.* (Unity Press, 1976)

Schor J. Emotions and health: Laughter really is good medicine. *Natural Medicine Journal.* 2010;2(1). Available at http://naturalmedicinejournal.com/article_content.asp?article=125.

CHAPTER 4

Chen X, Lu W, Zheng Y, et al. Exercise, tea consumption, and depression among breast cancer survivors. *J Clin Oncol.* 2010;28:991-998.

Duclos M, Corcuff JB, Pehourcq F, Tabarin A. Decreased pituitary sensitivity to glucocorticoids in endurance-trained men. *Eur J Endocrinol.* 2001;144:363-368.

Fairey AS, Courneya KS, Field CJ, Bell GJ, Jones LW, Mackey JR. Randomized controlled trial of exercise and blood immune function in postmenopausal breast cancer survivors. *J Appl Physiol.* 2005;98(4):1534-1540.

Martins RA, Verissimo MT, Coelho e Silva MJ, Cumming SP, Teixeira AM. Effects of aerobic and strength-based training on metabolic health indicators in older adults. *Lipids Health Dis.* 2010;9:76-82.

Musto A, Jacobs K, Nash M, DelRossi G, Perry A. The effects of an incremental approach to 10,000 steps/day on metabolic syndrome components in sedentary overweight women. *Phys Act Health.* 2010;7(6):737-745.

Rikli RE, Jones CJ. Development and validation of a functional fitness test for community-residing older adults. *J Aging Phys Activ.* 1999;7:129-161.

Rogers CJ, Colbert LH, Greiner JW, Perkins SN, Hursting SD. Physical activity and cancer prevention : pathways and targets for intervention. *Sports Med.* 2008;38(4):271-296.

Ryan AS. Insulin resistance with aging: effects of diet and exercise. *Sports Med.* 2000;30(5):327-346.

Stookey JD, Constant F, Popkin BM, Gardner CD. Drinking water is associated with weight loss in overweight dieting women independent of diet and activity. *Obesity.* 2008;16(11):2481-2488.

Taylor-Piliae RE, Haskell WL, Stotts NA, Froelicher ES. Improvement in balance, strength, and flexibility after 12 weeks of Tai chi exercise in ethnic Chinese adults with cardiovascular disease risk factors. *Altern Ther Health Med.* 2006;12(2):50-58.

CHAPTER 5

Aggarwal B, Shishodia S. Molecular targets of dietary agents for prevention and therapy of cancer. *Biochem Pharmacol.* 2006;71:1397-1421.

Anand P, Kunnumakara A, Sundaram C, et al. Cancer is a preventable disease that requires major lifestyle changes. *Pharm Res.* 2008;25(9):2097-2116.

Beasley JM, Newcomb PA, Trentham-Dietz A, et al. Post-diagnosis dietary factors and survival after invasive breast cancer. *Breast Cancer Res Treat.* 2011 Jan 1. [Epub ahead of print]

Bhatia E, Doddivenaka C, Zhang X, et al. Chemopreventive effects of dietary canola oil on colon cancer development. *Nutr Cancer.* 2011;63(2):242-247.

Camargo A, Ruano J, Fernandez JM, et al. Gene expression changes in mononuclear cells in patients with metabolic syndrome after acute intake of phenol-rich virgin olive oil. *BMC Genomics.* 2010;11:253.

Castillo-Pichardo L, Martínez-Montemayor MM, Martínez JE, Wall KM, Cubano LA, Dharmawardhane S. Inhibition of mammary tumor growth and metastases to bone and liver by dietary grape polyphenols. *Clin Exp Metastasis*. 2009;26(6):505-516.

Guha N, Kwan M, Quesenberry Jr C, Weltzien E. Soy isoflavones and risk of cancer recurrence in a cohort of breast cancer survivors: the Life After Cancer Epidemiology study. *Breast Cancer Res Treat*. 2009;118(2):395-405.

Gunter M, Hoover D, Yu H, et al. Insulin, insulin-like growth factor-1, and risk of breast cancer in postmenopausal women. *J Natl Cancer Inst*. 2009;101:48-60.

Karlsen A, Retterstøl L, Laake P, et al. Anthocyanins inhibit nuclear factor-kappaB activation in monocytes and reduce plasma concentrations of pro-inflammatory mediators in healthy adults. *J Nutr*. 2007;137(8):1951-1954.

Kayashima T, Mori M, Yoshida H, Mizushina Y, Matsubara K. 1,4-Naphthoquinone is a potent inhibitor of human cancer cell growth and angiogenesis. *Cancer Lett*. 2009;278(1):34-40.

Liu RH. Potential synergy of phytochemicals in cancer prevention: mechanism of action. *J Nutr*. 2004;134:3479S-3485S.

Marquart L, Wiemer L, Jones J, Jacob B. Whole grains health claims in the USA and other efforts to increase whole-grain consumption. *Proc Nutr Soc*. 2003;62:151-160.

Martin K. Targeting apoptosis with dietary bioactive agents. *Exp Biol Med*. 2006;231:117-129.

McAfee AJ, McSorley EM, Cuskelly GJ, et al. Red meat from animals offered a grass diet increases plasma and platelet n-3 PUFA in healthy consumers. *Br J Nutr*. 2011;105(1):80-89.

McCullough M, Patel A, Kushi L, et al. Following cancer prevention guidelines reduces risk of cancer, cardiovascular disease and all-cause mortality. *Cancer Epidemiol Biomarkers Prev*. 2011 May 17. [Epub ahead of print]

Pérez-Jiménez J, Neveu V, Vos F, Scalbert A. Identification of the 100 richest dietary sources of polyphenols: an application of the Phenol-Explorer database. *Eur J Clin Nutr*. 2010;64(S3):S112-S120.

Rosa A, Shizgal H. The Harris Benedict equation re-evaluated: resting energy requirements and the body cell mass. *Am J Clin Nutr*. 1984;40:168-182.

Schutze M, Boeing H, Pischon T, et al. Alcohol attributable burden of incidence of cancer in eight European countries based on results from prospective cohort study. *Br Med J*. 2011;342:d1584.

Shu XO, Zheng Y, Cai H, et al. Soy food intake and breast cancer survival. *JAMA*. 2009;302(22):2437-2443.

Spadafranca A, Martinez Conesa C, Sirini S, Testolin G. Effect of dark chocolate on plasma epicatechin levels, DNA resistance to oxidative stress and total antioxidant activity in healthy subjects. *Br J Nutr*. 2010;103(7):1008-1014.

Stull AJ, Cash KC, Johnson WD, Champagne CM, Cefalu WT. Bioactives in blueberries improve insulin sensitivity in obese, insulin-resistant men and women. *J Nutr*. 2010;140(10):1764-1768.

van Dijk SJ, Feskens EJ, Bos MB, et al. A saturated fatty acid-rich diet induces an obesity-linked proinflammatory gene expression profile in adipose tissue of subjects at risk of metabolic syndrome. *Am J Clin Nutr*. 2009;90(6):1656-1664.

Villasenor A, Ambs A, Ballard-Barbash R, et al. Dietary fiber is associated with circulating concentrations of C-reactive protein in breast cancer survivors: the HEAL study. *Breast Cancer Res Treat.* 2011 Apr 1. [Epub ahead of print]

CHAPTER 6

Bertini G, Colavito V, Tognoli C, Etet PF, Bentivoglio M. The aging brain, neuroinflammatory signaling and sleep-wake regulation. *Ital J Anat Embryol.* 2010;115(1-2):31-38.

Dibner C, Schibler U, Albrecht U. The mammalian circadian timing system: organization and coordination of central and peripheral clocks. *Annu Rev Physiol.* 2010;72:517-549.

Donga E, van Dijk M, van Dijk JG, et al. A single night of partial sleep deprivation induces insulin resistance in multiple metabolic pathways in healthy subjects. *J Clin Endocrinol Metab.* 2010;95(6):2963-2968.

Duez H, Staels B. Rev-erb-alpha: an integrator of circadian rhythms and metabolism *J Appl Physiol.* 2009;107(6):1972-1980.

Faraut B, Boudjeltia KZ, Dyzma M, et al. Benefits of napping and an extended duration of recovery sleep on alertness and immune cells after acute sleep restriction. *Brain Behav Immun.* 2011;25(1):16-24.

Irwin M. Effects of sleep and sleep loss on immunity and cytokines. *Brain Behav Immun.* 2002;16(5):503-512.

Kryger MH, Mignot E, Orr WC, Ryan D, Walsh JK. National Sleep Foundation. Sleep in America Poll, 2002.

Mullington JM, Simpson NS, Meier-Ewert HK, Haack M. Sleep loss and inflammation. *Best Pract Res Clin Endocrinol Metab.* 2010;24(5):775-784.

Nosek M, Kennedy HP, Beyene Y, Taylor D, Gilliss C, Lee K. The effects of perceived stress and attitudes toward menopause and aging on symptoms of menopause. *J Midwifery Womens Health.* 2010;55(4):328-334.

Rafalson L, Donahue RP, Stranges S, et al. Short sleep duration is associated with the development of impaired fasting glucose: the Western New York Health Study. *Ann Epidemiol.* 2010;20(12):883-889.

Shurlygina AV, Mitshurina SV, Verbitskaja LV, et al. Structure of nuclear chromatin in cells of lymphoid organs and blood from mice maintained under abnormal light-dark cycle and treated with benz(a)pyrene. *Bull Exp Biol Med.* 2010;149(1):29-32.

Wynn E, Krieg MA, Aeschlimann JM, Burckhardt P. Alkaline mineral water lowers bone resorption even in calcium sufficiency: alkaline mineral water and bone metabolism. *Bone.* 2009;44(1):120-124.

Wynn E, Krieg MA, Lanham-New SA, Burckhardt P. Postgraduate Symposium: Positive influence of nutritional alkalinity on bone health. *Proc Nutr Soc.* 2010;69(1):166-173.

Zaharna M, Guilleminault C. Sleep, noise and health: review. *Noise Health.* 2010;12(47):64-69.

CHAPTER 7

Ahonen MH, Tenkanen L, Teppo L, Hakama M, Tuohimaa P. Prostate cancer risk and prediagnostic serum 25-hydroxyvitamin D levels (Finland). *Cancer Causes Control.* 2000;11(9):847-852.

Antony B, Merina B, Iyer V, et al. A pilot cross-over study to evaluate human oral bio-availability of BCM-95® CG (BiocurcumaxTM), a novel bioenhanced preparation of curcumin. *Indian J Pharm Sci.* 2008;70(4):445-450.

Athar M, Back JH, Tang X, et al. Resveratrol: a review of pre-clinical studies for human cancer prevention. *Appl Pharmacol.* 2007;224(3):274-283.

Bartoli GM, Palozza P, Marra G, et al. n-3 PUFA and alpha-tocopherol control of tumor cell proliferation. *Mol Aspects Med.* 1993;14(3):247-252.

Bettuzzi S, Brausi M, Rizzi F, et al. Chemoprevention of human prostate cancer by oral administration of green tea catechins in volunteers with high-grade prostate intraepithelial neoplasia: a preliminary report from a one-year proof-of-principle study. *Cancer Res.* 2006;66(2):1234-1240.

Black HS, Rhodes LE. The potential of omega-3 fatty acids in the prevention of non-melanoma skin cancer. *Cancer Detect Prev.* 2006;30(3):224-232.

Bocle J-C, Thomann C. Effects of probiotics and probiotics on flora and immunity in adults. *Agence Francaise de Securite Sanitaire des Aliments.* 2005:63-111.

Boge T, Rémigy M, Vaudaine S, Tanguy J, Bourdet-Sicard R, van der Werf S. A probiotic fermented dairy drink improves antibody response to influenza vaccination in the elderly in two randomised controlled trials. *Vaccine.* 2009;27(41):5677-5684.

Boocock DJ, Faust GE, Patel KR, et al. Phase I dose escalation pharmacokinetic study in healthy volunteers of resveratrol, a potential cancer chemopreventive agent. *Cancer Epidemiol Biomarkers Prev.* 2007;16(6):1246-1252.

Brown VA, Patel KR, Viskaduraki M, et al. Repeat dose study of the cancer chemopreventive agent resveratrol in healthy volunteers: safety, pharmacokinetics, and effect on the insulin-like growth factor axis. *Cancer Res.* 2010;70(22):9003-9011.

Cani PD, Delzenne NM. Interplay between obesity and associated metabolic disorders: new insights into the gut microbiota. *Curr Opinion Pharmacol.* 2009;9:737-743.

Carpenter DO. Environmental contaminants as risk factors for developing diabetes. *Rev Environ Health.* 2008;23(1):59-74.

Chen Y, Tseng SH. Review. Pro- and anti-angiogenesis effects of resveratrol. *In Vivo.* 2007;21(2):365-370.

Cheng AL, Hsu CH, Lin JK, et al. Phase I clinical trial of curcumin, a chemopreventive agent, in patients with high-risk or pre-malignant lesions. *Anticancer Res.* 2001;21:2895-2900.

Chiu A, Chan JL, Kern DG, Kohler S et al. Double-blinded, placebo-controlled trial of green tea extracts in the clinical and histologic appearance of photoaging skin. *Dermatol Surg.* 2005;31:855-859.

Cuomo J, Appendino G, Dern AS, et al. Comparative absorption of a standardized curcuminoid mixture and its lecithin formulation. *J Nat Prod.* 2011;74(4):664-669.

Cruz-Correa M, Shoskes D, Sanches P, et al. Combination treatment with curcumin and quercetin of adenomas in familial adenomatous polyposis. *Clin Gastroenterol Hepatol.* 2006;4:1035-1038.

de Vrese M, Winkler P, Rautenberg P, et al. Effect of Lactobacillus gasseri PA 16/8, Bifidobacterium longum SP 07/3, B. bifidum MF 20/5 on common cold episodes: a double blind, randomized, controlled trial. *Clin Nutr.* 2005;24(4):481-491.

Eastwood GL. Pharmacologic prevention of colonic neoplasms. Effects of calcium, vitamins, omega fatty acids, and nonsteroidal anti-inflammatory drugs. *Dig Dis.* 1996;14(2):119-128.

Enyeart JA, Liu H, Enyeart JJ. Curcumin inhibits ACTH- and angiotensin II-stimulated cortisol secretion and Ca(v)3.2 current. *J Nat Prod.* 2009;72(8):1533-1537.

Fedirko V, Bostick RM, Flanders WD, et al. Effects of vitamin D and calcium supplementation on markers of apoptosis in normal colon mucosa: A randomized, double-blind, placebo-controlled clinical trial. *Can Prev Res.* 2009;2(3)213-223.

Gao YT, McLaughlin JK, Blot WJ, et al. Reduced risk of esophageal cancer associated with green tea consumption. *J Natl Cancer Inst.* 1994;86(11):855-858.

Gago-Dominquez M, Castelao E, Sun C-L, et al. Marine n-3 fatty acid intake, glutathione S-transferase polymorphisms and breast cancer risk in postmenopausal Chinese women in Singapore. *Carcinogenesis.* 2004;25(11):2143-2147.

Garland C, Grant W, Mohr S, et al. What is the dose-response relationship between vitamin D and cancer risk? *Nutr Rev.* 2007;65(8):S91-S95.

Goodwin PJ, Ennis M, Pritchard KI, Koo J, Hood N. Prognostic effects of 25-hydroxyvitamin D levels in early breast cancer. *J Clin Oncol.* 2009;27(23):3757-3763.

Gorham ED, Garland CF, Garland FC, et al. Optimal vitamin D status for colorectal cancer prevention: a quantitative meta analysis. *Am J Prev Med.* 2007;32(3):210-216.

Heller AR, Rössel T, Gottschlich B, et al. Omega-3 fatty acids improve liver and pancreas function in postoperative cancer patients. *Int J Cancer.* 2004;111(4):611-616.

Holub B, Hoffer LJ, Jones P. Clinical nutrition: 4. Omega-3 fatty acids in cardiovascular care. *Canadian Med Assoc Journal.* 2002;166(5):608-615.

Inoue M, Tajima K, Mizutani M, et al. Regular consumption of green tea and the risk of breast cancer recurrence: follow-up study from the Hospital-based Epidemiologic Research Program at Aichi Cancer Center (HERPACC), Japan. *Cancer Lett.* 2001;167(2):175-182.

Ishikawa H, Akedo I, Otani T, et al. Randomized trial of dietary fiber and Lactobacillus casei administration for prevention of colorectal tumors. *Int J Cancer.* 2005;116(5):762-767.

Iwasaki M, Inoue M, Sasazuki S, et al. Green tea drinking and subsequent risk of breast cancer in a population based cohort of Japanese women. *Breast Cancer Res.* 2010;12:R88

Joe AK, Liu H, Suzui M, Vural ME, Xiao D, Weinstein IB. Resveratrol induces growth inhibition, S-phase arrest, apoptosis, and changes in biomarker expression in several human cancer cell lines. *Clin Cancer Res.* 2002;8(3):893-903.

John EM, Koo J, Schwartz GG. Sun exposure and prostate cancer risk: evidence for a protective effect of early-life exposure. *Cancer Epidemiol Biomarkers Prev.* 2007;16(6):1283-1286.

Kajander K, Myllyluoma E, Rajilić-Stojanović M, et al. Clinical trial: multispecies probiotic supplementation alleviates the symptoms of irritable bowel syndrome and stabilizes intestinal microbiota. *Aliment Pharmacol Ther.* 2008;27(1):48-57.

Kumar M, Kumar A, Nagpal R, et al. Cancer-preventing attributes of probiotics: an update. *Int J Food Sci Nutr.* 2010;61(5):473-496.

Kunnumakkara A, Guha S, Aggarwal B. Curcumin and colorectal cancer: add spice to your life. *Curr Colorectal Cancer Rep.* 2009;5:5-14.

la Porte C, Voduc N, Zhang G, et al. Steady-State pharmacokinetics and tolerability of trans-resveratrol 2000 mg twice daily with food, quercetin and alcohol (ethanol) in healthy human subjects. *Clin Pharmacokinet.* 2010;49(7):449-454.

Lappe JM, Travers-Gustafson D, Davies KM, Recker RR, Heaney RP. Vitamin D and calcium supplementation reduces cancer risk; results of a randomized trial. *Am J Clin Nutr.* 2007;85:1586-1591.

Li Y-H, Wu Y, Wei HC, et al. Protective effects of green tea extracts on photoaging and photoimmunosuppression. *Skin Res Technology.* 2009;15:338-345.

Mawer E, Walls J, Howell A, et al. Serum 1,25-dihydroxyvitamin D may be related inversely to disease activity in breast cancer patients with bone metastases. *J Clin Endocrinol Metab.* 1997;82:118-122.

Nakachi K, Suemasu K, Suga K, Takeo T, Imai K, Higashi Y. Influence of drinking green tea on breast cancer malignancy among Japanese patients. *Jpn J Cancer Res.* 1998;89(3):254-261.

Nantz M, Rowe CA, Bukowski JF, Percival SS. Standardized capsule of Camellia sinensis lowers cardiovascular risk factors in a randomized, double-blind, placebo controlled study. *Nutrition.* 2009;25:147-154.

Narayanan BA, Narayanan NK, Re GG, Nixon DW. Differential expression of genes induced by resveratrol in LNCaP cells: P53-mediated molecular targets. *Int J Cancer.* 2003;104(2):204-212.

National Health and Nutrition Examination Survey. What we eat in America, 2005-2006. Available at: http://www.ars.usda.gov/ba/bhnrc/fsrg. Accessed May 23, 2011.

Ouwehand AC, Bergsma N, Parhiala R, et al. Bifidobacterium microbiota and parameters of immune function in elderly subjects. *FEMS Immunol Med Microbiol.* 2008;53(1):18-25.

Patel KR, Brown VA, Jones DJ, et al. Clinical pharmacology of resveratrol and its metabolites in colorectal cancer patients. *Cancer Res.* 2010;70(19):7392-7399.

Prucksunand C, Indrasukhsri B, Leethochawalit M, Hungspreugs K. Phase II clinical trial on effect of the long turmeric (*Curcuma longa* Linn) on healing of peptic ulcer. *Southeast Asian J Trop Med Public Health.* 2001;32:208-215.

Puertollano MA, Puertollano E, de Cienfuegos GA, de Pablo MA. Dietary antioxidants: immunity and host defense. *Curr Top Med Chem.* 2011 Apr 21. [Epub ahead of print]

Rosen C. Vitamin D insufficiency. *N Engl J Med.* 2011;364:248-254.

Setiawan VW, Zhang ZF, Yu GP, et al. Protective effect of green tea on the risks of chronic gastritis and stomach cancer. *Int J Cancer.* 2001;92(4):600-604.

Shimizu M, Fukutomi Y, Ninomiya M, et al. Green tea extracts for the prevention of metachronous colorectal adenomas: a pilot study. *Cancer Epid Biomarkers Prev.* 2008;17(11):3020-3025.

Showell MG, Brown J, Yazdani A, Stankiewicz MT, Hart RJ. Antioxidants for male subfertility. *Cochrane Database Syst Rev.* 2011;(1):CD007411.

Walle T, Hsieh F, DeLegge MH, Oatis JE Jr, Walle UK. High absorption but very low bioavailability of oral resveratrol in humans. *Drug Metab Dispos.* 2004;32(12):1377-1382.

Wu M, Harvey KA, Ruzmetov N, et al. Omega-3 polyunsaturated fatty acids attenuate breast cancer growth through activation of a neutral sphingomyelinase-mediated pathway. *Int J Cancer.* 2005;117(3):340-348.

Zeng J, Li YQ, Zuo XL, Zhen YB, Yang J, Liu CH. Clinical trial: effect of active lactic acid bacteria on mucosal barrier function in patients with diarrhoea-predominant irritable bowel syndrome. *Aliment Pharmacol Ther.* 2008;28(8):994-1002.

Zou J, Dong J, Yu X. Meta-analysis: Lactobacillus containing quadruple therapy versus standard triple first-line therapy for Helicobacter pylori eradication. *Helicobacter.* 2009;14(5):97-107.

CHAPTER 8

Andrew MD, et al. American Cancer Society guidelines for early detection of prostate cancer: Update 2010. *CA Cancer J Clin.* 2010;60:70-98.

Cunningham D, et al. Colorectal cancer. *Lancet.* 2010;375:1030-1047.

Drazer MW, et al. Population-based patterns and predictors of prostate-specific antigen screening among older men in the United States. *J Clin Oncol.* 2011;29(13):1763-1743.

Elit L, et al. Follow-up for women after treatment for cervical cancer. *Curr Oncol.* 2010;17(3):65-69.

Kulie T, et al. Obesity and women's health: An evidence-based review. *J Am Board Fam Med.* 2011;24:75-85.

Kurman RJ, et al. Early detection and treatment of ovarian cancer: shifting from early stage to minimal volume of disease based on a new model of carcinogenesis. *Am J Obstet Gynecol.* 2008;198(4):351-356.

Robbins CL, et al . Influence of reproductive factors on mortality after epithelial ovarian cancer diagnosis. *Cancer Epidemiol Biomarkers Prev.* 2009;18(7):2035-2041.

Salhab M, Bismohun S, Mokbel K. Risk-reducing strategies for women carrying BRCA1/2 mutations with a focus on prophylactic surgery. *BMC Womens Health.* 2010;10-28.

Sandblom G, et al. Randomized prostate cancer screening trial: 20 year follow-up. *BMJ.* 2011;342:d1539.

Winchester DP. Post-treatment surveillance of breast cancer patients in an organized, multidisciplinary setting. *J Surg Oncol.* 2011;103(4):358-361.

Wong EM, et al. Constitutional methylation of the BRCA1 promoter is specifically associated with BRCA1 mutation-associated pathology in early-onset breast cancer. *Cancer Prev Res.* 2011;4(1):23-33.

CHAPTER 9

Clodi M, et al. Oxytocin alleviates the neuroendocrine and cytokine response to bacterial endotoxin in healthy men. *Am J Physiol Endodrinol Metab.* 2008;295(3):E686-F691.

Corporation for National and Community Service. Volunteering produces health benefits. Available at: http://www.nationalservice.gov/about/newsroom/releases_detail.asp?tbl_pr_id=687. Accessed April 18, 2011.

Grimm R, Spring K, Dietz N. The health benefits of volunteering: a review of recent research. Corporation for National and Community Service Report. April 2007.

Parkinson L, Warburton J, Sibbritt D, Byles J. Volunteering and older women: psychosocial and health predictors of participation. *Aging Ment Health.* 2010;14(8):917-927.

Remen RN. Soul work: Integrating the spirit in healthcare. Integrative Healthcare Symposium. New York City. March 6, 2011.

Remen RN. Personal correspondence. May 2011.

INDEX

ABOUT THE AUTHORS

DR. LISE ALSCHULER is a practicing naturopathic physician with board certification in naturopathic oncology. Dr. Alschuler has been in practice since 1994. She is past President of the American Association of Naturopathic Physicians. Dr. Alschuler is the Vice President of Quality and Education at Emerson Ecologics in Bedford, New Hampshire, the leading provider of professional-grade nutritional supplements, products, and services to the integrative healthcare community. She provides naturopathic oncology consultations through Naturopathic Specialists LLC at Northeast Integrative Medicine in Bedford, NH.

Dr. Alschuler graduated from Brown University in 1988 with an undergraduate degree in Medical Anthropology. In 1994, she received her doctorate of naturopathic medicine from Bastyr University. As a clinical associate professor, Dr. Alschuler has taught botanical medicine, gastroenterology, and clinical skills to naturopathic students. She was founding Chair of the Botanical Medicine program at Southwest College of Naturopathic Medicine in Scottsdale, AZ, and later Chair of the Botanical Medicine department at Bastyr University in Kenmore, WA. She then became medical director of the Bastyr University outpatient clinic. In 2003, she became the director of the naturopathic medicine department at Cancer Treatment Centers of America—Midwestern Regional Medical Center in greater Chicago, IL, where she managed naturopathic oncology care and program development provided at this 95-bed JCAHO accredited regional hospital.

Dr. Alschuler is on the boards of the American Board of Naturopathic Oncology Medical Examiners and the Naturopathic Post-Graduate Association, and was a founding board member of the Oncology Association of Naturopathic Physicians. She has published numerous articles on herbal medicine and naturopathic medicine in the lay press as well as in the medical literature. She co-authored a comprehensive guide for both the layperson and health professionals called *The Definitive Guide to Cancer: An Integrative Approach to Prevention, Treatment and Healing* (3rd edition, Random House, 2010). She has lectured extensively on these topics nationally as well as internationally. In September 2000 she was named by Seattle Magazine as one of Seattle's Top Doctors.

KAROLYN A. GAZELLA began her career in journalism working at a newspaper, radio station, and then local television. She started her first consulting business when she was 26 years old. She has worked in the natural health industry in both marketing and publishing since 1992. She is the founding publisher of the peer-reviewed journal *Integrative Medicine* and has written hundreds of articles for both consumers and healthcare professionals. She is the co-author of *The Definitive Guide to Cancer, Boost Your Health With Bacteria,* and *Return to Beautiful Skin.* She is also the creator and managing editor of the Healthy Living Guide Series of booklets and books available through Active Interest Media, publishers of *Yoga Journal, Vegetarian Times, Better Nutrition, Amazing Wellness,* and many other quality magazines. Karolyn is the founder and publisher of *Natural Medicine Journal,* an innovative peer-reviewed e-journal and open access website (www.naturalmedicinejournal.com). In 2009 she was recognized by the Integrator Blog as one of the "Top 10 People in Integrative Health Care and Integrative Medicine."